LAMBTON COUNTY LIBRARY

2 0210 00734628 2

D1370910

DATE DUE			

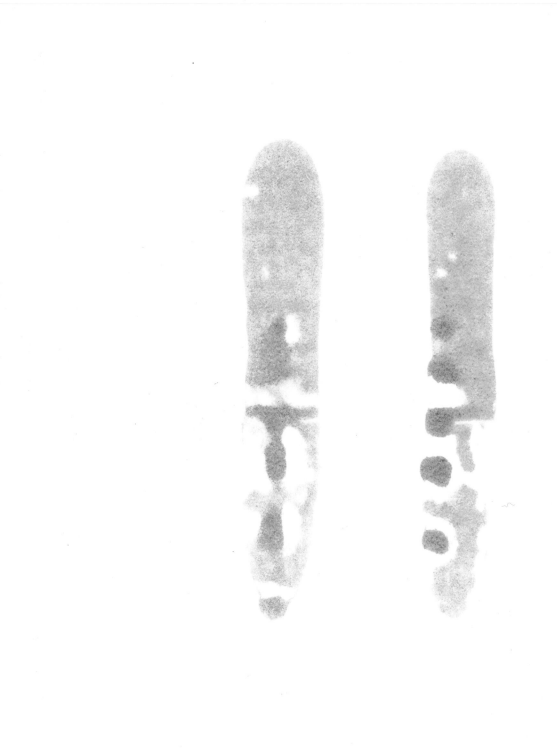

Super Firm

Tough Workouts

EDITORIAL BOARD OF ADVISORS

Eva S. Auchincloss, Consultant, Women's Sports Foundation

Dorothy V. Harris, Ph.D., Professor, Laboratory for Human Performance Research, The Pennsylvania State University; U.S. Olympic Sports Psychology Advisory Committee

Hans Howald, M.D., Professor, Biochemistry of Exercise, Swiss National Training Institute, Magglingen, Switzerland

Paavo V. Komi, Ph.D., Professor, Department of Biology of Physical Activity, University of Jyvaskyla, Finland

Joyce C. Lashof, M.D., Dean, School of Public Health, University of California, Berkeley

Joyce T. Leung, R.D., MS., M.P.H., Department of Pediatrics, Columbia University

William D. McArdle, Ph.D., Professor, Department of Health and Physical Education, Queens College

Sheldon Margen, M.D., Professor, Department of Public Health Nutrition, University of California, Berkeley

Jeffrey Minkoff, M.D., Director, Sports Medicine Center, New York University

Mitsumasa Miyashita, Ph.D., Professor, Laboratory for Exercise Physiology and Biomechanics, Tokyo University, Japan; Fellow, American College of Sports Medicine

Richard C. Nelson, Ph.D., Director, Biomechanics Laboratory, The Pennsylvania State University

Benno M. Nigg, Ph.D., Director, Laboratory for Human Performance Studies, Faculty of Physical Education, University of Calgary

Ralph S. Paffenbarger Jr., M.D., Professor of Epidemiology, Department of Family, Community and Preventive Medicine, Stanford University School of Medicine

Allan J. Ryan, M.D., Director, Sports Medicine Enterprise; former Editor-in-Chief, The Physician and Sportsmedicine

Bengt Saltin, M.D., Ph.D., Professor, August Krogh Institute, University of Copenhagen, Denmark

Christine L. Wells, Ph.D., Professor, Department of Health and Physical Education, Arizona State University

Myron Winick, M.D., R.R. Williams Professor of Nutrition, Institute of Human Nutrition, College of Physicians and Surgeons, Columbia University

William B. Zuti, Ph.D., Director, Pepsico Fitness Center; Fellow, American College of Sports Medicine; former national director of health enhancement, YMCA

Super Firm

Tough Workouts

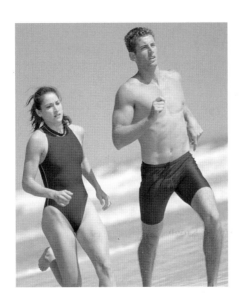

TIME®
LIFE

by the Editors of Time-Life Books

LAMBTON COUNTY LIBRARY, WYOMING, ONTARIO

CONSULTANTS FOR THIS BOOK

William D. McArdle, Ph.D., is a professor in the Department of Health and Physical Education at Queens College of the City University of New York. A Fellow of the American College of Sports Medicine, he is the author of *Exercise Physiology: Energy, Nutrition, and Human Performance; Getting in Shape* and *Nutrition, Weight Control, and Exercise.*

Robert Panariello, M.S., a registered physical therapist, certified athletic trainer, and certified strength and conditioning specialist, is a senior physical therapist at the Sportsmedicine Performance and Research center, Hospital for Special Surgery, in New York City. He is also the strength and conditioning coordinator for the St. John's University basketball team, and has served as an athletic trainer at the Olympic Training Center in Lake Placid, New York.

Ann Piccarillo is the owner and director of Manhattan Body, Inc., an exercise studio in New York City. She is a member of the Reebok Advisory Board and is certified by the Aerobics and Fitness Association of America.

Bonnie Bennett Stauffer, Ed.D., is the Director of Upperclass Physical Education at the United States Military Academy at West Point, New York, and serves as an instructor in the Master Fitness Trainer Program for the United States Army. Stauffer has also served as the sports psychologist for the Canadian National Wrestling Team.

Nutritional Consultants

Ann Grandjean, Ed.D., is Associate Director of the Swanson Center for Nutrition, Omaha, Neb.; chief nutrition consultant to the U.S. Olympic Committee; and an instructor in the Sports Medicine Program, Orthopedic Surgery Department, University of Nebraska Medical Center.

Myron Winick, M.D., is the R.R. Williams Professor of Nutrition, Professor of Pediatrics, Director of the Institute of Human Nutrition, and Director of the Center for Nutrition, Genetics and Human Development at Columbia University College of Physicians and Surgeons. He has served on the Food and Nutrition Board of the National Academy of Sciences and is the author of many books, including *Your Personalized Health Profile.*

This edition published in 2005
by the Caxton Publishing Group
20 Bloomsbury Street, London WC1B 3JH

Under license from Time-Life Books BV.

Cover Design: Open Door Limited, Rutland UK

Title: Super Firm

ISBN: 1 84447 166 7

© 1989 Time Life Inc.

All rights reserved. No part of this book may be reproduced in any form or by any electronic or mechanical means, including information storage and retrieval devices or systems, without prior written permission from the copyright owner, except that brief passages may be quoted for reviews.

TIME-LIFE is a registered trademark of Time Warner Inc. and affiliated companies. Used under license.

Some of the exercises in this book are advanced and should not be attempted by anyone who is not already physically fit. This book is not intended as a substitute for the advice of a physician or an athletic coach. Readers who have or suspect they may have specific medical problems should consult a physician before beginning any programme of strenuous physical exercise.

CONTENTS

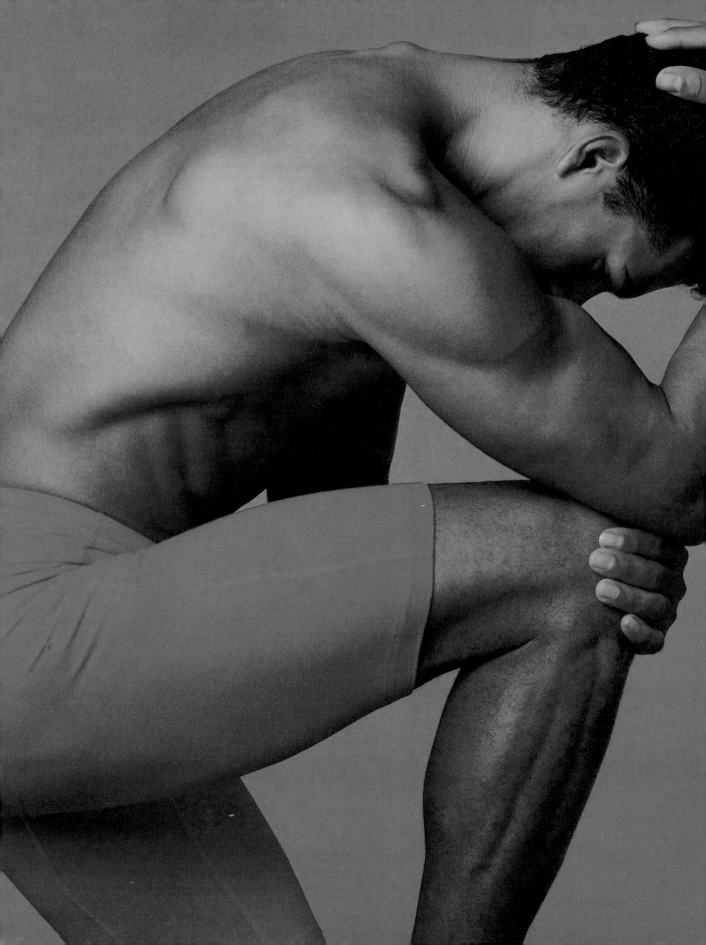

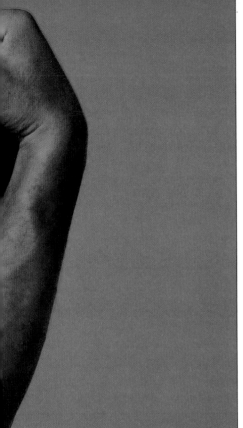

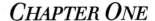
Working Harder

How to vary your exercise programme to enhance strength, power and muscle tone

I f building firm, well-toned muscles is your principal goal in exercising, it is not as if your selection of exercises is limited. There are dozens of different routines that can strengthen your muscles and help you mould a pleasingly contoured physique. Yet even well-conditioned people let their exercise programmes lapse at times for a simple reason: performing the same routines again and again can become monotonous, and you arrive at a point where your level of fitness reaches a plateau and you no longer see much physical improvement.

This book is designed to revitalize your exercise programme by presenting a series of harder-than-average workouts that have been designed to require little or no equipment, and — as this chapter explains — that offer quite distinctive ways of taxing or overloading your muscles. Some are advanced variations on familiar muscle-strengthening callisthenic routines; others show new ways to sequence exercises in a manner that makes the total workout more demanding to perform; and, finally, there are techniques for developing power, an aspect of fitness related to muscle strength and tone.

What gives muscles firmness and shape?

Truly firm muscles have both strength, which involves the maximum exertion of a single contraction, and endurance, or the ability to perform repeated contractions. These elements are interrelated: a soccer player needs muscular endurance to run the length of the field; he also needs power to perform the single, explosive effort to kick or head a ball. The only way to build muscular strength and endurance is to force the muscles to bear some kind of load, which is called resistance. This resistance can take the form of free weights or weight machines, or you can lift the weight of your body, as in a push-up or sit-up.

Both lifting your body weight and exercising with an external load stress your muscles in an identical way, causing them to contract and begin a complex series of chemical reactions. This results in changes in the enzymes responsible for fat metabolism, and in the number and size of mitochondria — the cell structures responsible for the release of energy — and numerous other improvements. The more you exercise your muscles at or near maximum capacity, the more they adapt: they grow in strength, and to some degree in size as well.

Can callisthenics that do not use weights provide a sufficiently strenuous workout?

Callisthenics affect not just the primary muscle groups they target, but also the muscles that assist the movement by stabilizing the body. In a push-up exercise, for example, the up-and-down motion works your arms, chest and shoulders directly. However, your abdominals, thighs, hip flexors, back muscles and buttocks are also given a workout, if less intensely, by their role in keeping the body rigid during the movement. Physiologists refer to this secondary level of toning as muscle co-contraction. By contrast, weight training — particularly with the use of machines — tends to pinpoint individual muscle groups, and there is less co-contraction by assisting muscles.

Do exercises that rely solely on your body weight allow you to adjust the resistance?

Weight training does offer one major advantage over callisthenics. Because weight can easily be added to or subtracted, it is easier to regulate the resistance you are working with precisely, and to increase it as you progress. The incremental progression of the load is a basic training method called progressive resistance. This concept is based on research showing that to build strength you must keep resistance high and the number of repetitions low — simply adding reps will build local muscular endurance but not strength. In effect, if you can easily perform an exercise more than 10 times in succession, you must increase the load in order to best achieve additional strength gains.

A major goal in beginning a muscle-building programme is to improve your physique, and there are sound psychological reasons behind this impulse. A study of 142 male college students found that the stronger, more muscularly fit among them had a significantly better self-image than their peers. The stronger men were shown in psychological tests to be more confident, emotionally stable and outgoing than the others.

EASY

MEDIUM

HARD

● Centre of gravity
● Axis of movement

Making an Exercise Harder

As you grow stronger and your muscles get accustomed to working out, the initial exercises in your strength-training programme will become too easy: they no longer provide enough resistance for your muscles to contract against, and if you do not increase the weight, your strength gains will start to level off. The key to increasing the load lies in the mechanics of movement, as shown in the illustrations.

In the sit-up, for example, you move your torso from the hips (the axis of movement). The weight of your torso (applied through the centre of gravity) resists this movement. If you can add more weight at this point, the resistance will be greater — and the exercise will therefore be more difficult.

The sit-up shown in the top illustration, with your arms extended at your sides, is the easiest to perform because the centre of gravity is fairly low in your chest. The result is less weight to hoist. Placing your arms on your chest (*centre*), or at the side of your head covering your ears (*bottom*), has the effect of moving the centre of gravity upwards. This means you must lift and lower more weight, as suggested by the increasing size of the triangles in the illustrations, effectively creating additional overload.

How Plyometrics Improves Performance

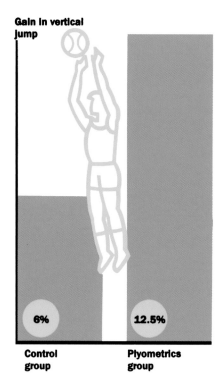

Gain in vertical jump

6%

Control group

12.5%

Plyometrics group

The bounding and jumping drills in plyometrics are used by many sports teams to build a type of strength that is ignored by most training programmes: "explosive" power. In one study of university basketball players, the group that added plyometrics to its training regimens showed a far more significant increase in vertical jump heights than the control group, as shown above.

Although you cannot control resistance as rigorously when you are relying on your own body weight, the load of an exercise can nevertheless be adjusted by variations in the way that the movement is performed. By changing the angle of your body position or shifting your centre of gravity, you can advance to increasingly more difficult versions of standard exercises, as shown in the illustrations on page 9. For example, by performing one of the toughest push-up variations — the scapular shrug, with your torso suspended between two chairs — you greatly increase the load on your upper body muscles. Chapter Two focuses on this concept, offering exercise variations of increasing difficulty that will progressively improve your muscle strength and endurance as you become better conditioned.

Another way of adjusting the amount of stress you place on your muscles while exercising is regulating the pace at which you perform your workout — a technique that is the basis of the circuit-training routines presented in Chapter Four.

What is circuit training?

Developed in Great Britain, circuit training involves moving rapidly through a series of 15 to 20 exercises, or stations, targeting different body parts. The idea is to perform the activities consecutively, completing a given number of repetitions at each station but taking very little rest time between exercises. The vigorous pace serves two functions: it can be an effective way to achieve an overload effect, and it can also produce some aerobic, or cardiovascular, benefits along with firming and toning the specific muscles. This book presents a circuit-training routine adapted from a programme used at the United States Military Academy at West Point.

Does strength training also increase muscle power?

Technically, physiologists view muscle power as a subcomponent of strength that defines quick movements in which you propel your body weight upwards or forwards in short, "explosive" bursts of energy. The vertical jump and standing broad jump, for example, are both high-power activities. Since the force capacity of muscles in slow movements, such as callisthenics, gives some indication of force in quick action, strong muscles will generally be powerful as well. However, it is possible to supplement your training programme with routines designed to build explosive power, in addition to speed.

What is the best way to build power?

A relatively new form of exercise called plyometrics, which involves drills such as jumping, hopping and bounding, is being used by many professional athletes, including basketball and soccer players, tennis and squash players, divers, volleyball players, sprinters and others whose sports require short, intense bursts of activity. Plyometric movements rapidly force the muscles into two types of contractions consecutively: eccentric (lengthening against resistance) and concentric (shortening). The theory is that during the eccentric phase — for example, when you land after a jump — the combination of body weight and gravity creates a forceful contraction that loads your muscles with elastic energy. Then in the concentric phase — when you propel yourself into another jump, for instance — this energy is released in a powerful burst of kinetic (moving) energy, in much the same way as a rubber band shoots forwards when released after being stretched. Athletes are reporting success in building explosive power with plyometric drills. Chapter Three offers a complete plyometrics routine designed to condition you for high-power sports.

What happens if you stop training?

Just as muscles can always be developed, no matter how old you are, they can also deteriorate, regardless of your condition. Detraining — a loss in the ability to function — occurs in all skeletal muscles that are used less intensely than usual. If you have to wear a plaster cast on your leg, for example, your calf muscle will begin to become weaker and smaller, and you will have to exercise it specifically when the cast is removed to restore it to its normal appearance and capacity for work. Therefore, even if you are well conditioned, if you stop your workout programme completely, your muscle tone will disappear in about five to 10 weeks. In fact, former athletes who have not adopted exercise programmes are often in worse condition than nonathletes who play amateur sports consistently several times a week.

So even if your muscles are extremely firm and well conditioned, you must continue to exercise in order to maintain your strength and endurance, just as you must continue to perform an aerobic workout to maintain your cardiovascular fitness. The exercises in this book will not only help you to maintain your level of development, but will allow you to enhance it as well.

Will you reach a plateau in any long-term exercise programme?

Typically, the most noticeable physical improvements in any type of conditioning programme occur at the beginning, during the first few months. After that, your body continues to make incremental adaptations that are far less dramatic than your initial gains. At each stage, achieving additional development requires increasing your level of effort. After a while, you will arrive at a point where you are in good shape, and to keep pushing may not be possible — or may even result in an injury. Only you can determine your individual goals in an exercise programme and the appropriate time to ease off a bit and perform a routine that will maintain your physical condition. The self-assessment tests described on pages 12-13 will give you an idea of your current level of muscular fitness; the guidelines in the following chapters will help you determine the optimal exercises for you and the approximate length of your workout.

Sizing Yourself Up

The exercises in this book will help make your muscles very firm, whether you choose classic callisthenics (Chapter Two), a circuit-training programme (Chapter Four) or plyometric drills to build explosive power and enhance athletic performance (Chapter Three). Before you plunge into your exercise programme, take a few moments to assess your current level of strength.

The exercises on the opposite page will give you an indication of the strengths and weaknesses of your body. This knowledge will help you decide which exercise variations to include in your workout from those given in the following chapters. Jot down the number of repetitions you are able to perform in the four self-assessment tests and retest yourself every month or so to measure your improvement. This can be a powerful tool for self-motivation — and it can be very satisfying to see your muscle strength progress.

Whatever the routine you design for yourself, precede it with a five to 10-minute warm-up period and follow it with a five to 10-minute cool-down. The warm-up prepares your muscles and joints for exertion by increasing the blood flow and warming the tissues. This makes them less susceptible to strains and pulls. The cool-down helps speed recovery by removing lactic acid, a metabolic by-product that can cause pain or soreness if it accumulates in the muscles and bloodstream.

For best results, you should exercise three to five times a week and supplement your muscle routines with an aerobic workout three times a week. The aerobic activity, such as running, biking, swimming or circuit training, will build cardiovascular endurance, which — together with muscle strength — is the foundation of overall fitness.

To prevent fatigue, organize your workouts so that each muscle group gets a rest period between exercises. For instance, if you are performing two types of exercises to strengthen your abdominals, alternate them with movements for other body parts. Also, exercise the muscles that are more easily fatigued last: if you are weakest in the upper body, save your push-up sets for the end of your workout routine.

Score the tests as follows: Sit-ups: *Excellent* — 50; *Good* — 40; *Fair* — 30; Knee dips: *Excellent* — 20; *Good* — 15; *Fair* — 10; Push-ups: *Excellent* — 20; *Good* — 15; *Fair* — 10; Squat thrusts: *Excellent* — 20; *Good* — 15; *Fair* — 10.

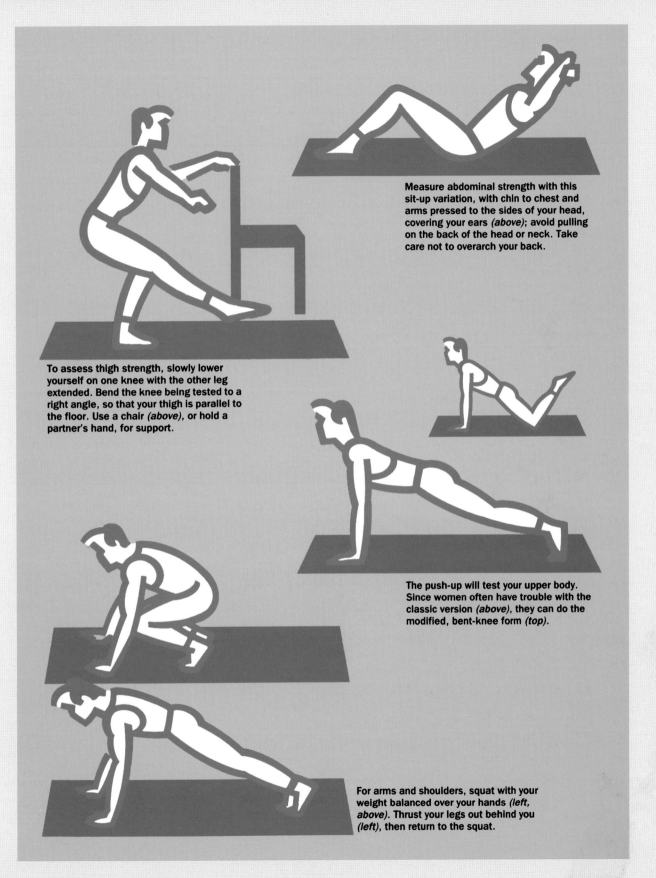

Measure abdominal strength with this sit-up variation, with chin to chest and arms pressed to the sides of your head, covering your ears *(above)*; avoid pulling on the back of the head or neck. Take care not to overarch your back.

To assess thigh strength, slowly lower yourself on one knee with the other leg extended. Bend the knee being tested to a right angle, so that your thigh is parallel to the floor. Use a chair *(above)*, or hold a partner's hand, for support.

The push-up will test your upper body. Since women often have trouble with the classic version *(above)*, they can do the modified, bent-knee form *(top)*.

For arms and shoulders, squat with your weight balanced over your hands *(left, above)*. Thrust your legs out behind you *(left)*, then return to the squat.

Myths of Power Eating

Are there foods that can make you stronger and more powerful or enhance your endurance? Many people believe that certain special substances — ranging from bee pollen to wheat germ — have powers that are almost magical. And for a number of years, athletes, trainers and even some scientists attributed strength-building properties to protein and recommended a diet that was high in protein and low in carbohydrates.

In fact, as the chart on pages 16-17 shows, foods that supposedly increase strength and physical performance have never been shown to accomplish this. Most of these foods do not fulfil any dietary requirements, and those that do are needed in relatively small amounts.

This is true even of protein. While muscle is made of protein, your need for it, even when you undertake a strenuous exercise programme, is no greater than what is found in any well-balanced diet — a daily maximum of about 11 per cent of your calories. Most often, foods that are relatively high in protein are also high in fat, a nutrient people in the West tend to get too much of. The chart opposite shows the relative percentage of carbohydrates and fat accompanying high-protein foods.

The list that follows details some common myths about protein.

Extra protein supplies additional energy, increases muscle mass and enhances athletic performance.

There is no evidence that increasing your protein intake above the Recommended Daily Amount will provide you with more energy, give you bigger and stronger muscles or improve your athletic performance. Nor do athletes require any more protein than their sedentary counterparts. Using your muscles does not cause them to deteriorate, so no extra protein is required to rebuild them.

Unlike both carbohydrates and fat, protein has a minor role as an energy source; it is used only when you exhaust your carbohydrate stores and easily mobilized fat reserves. Even then, protein is an inefficient fuel.

Taking protein supplements is an effective way of increasing your overall protein intake.

Protein supplements are harder to digest than protein-rich food, and when used as a replacement, they are potentially dangerous. They can cause severe dehydration and overwork your liver and kidneys. Excess protein also increases your excretion of the mineral calcium, which can cause bone loss and fractures.

Taking amino acid supplements will enhance performance and increase muscle mass.

Amino acids are the building blocks of protein, but taking supplements will neither enhance athletic performance nor build bigger muscles. Like protein supplements, they can cause health problems. Excessive intake of individual amino acids may cause calcium loss, gout, metabolic disorders, kidney strain and dehydration. Moreover, taking single amino acid supplements can interfere with the absorption of other essential amino acids.

What You Get with Protein

Food		Serving size	Calories	Per cent of calories		
				Protein	Fat	Carbohydrates
Bacon		3 rashers cooked	130	15	85	0
Beef	T-bone steak	100 g cooked	390	26	74	0
Bologna sausage		3 slices	195	16	83	1
Bread	wholemeal	1 slice	60	12	15	73
Cheese	Cheddar	30 g	120	25	74	1
	cottage, 4% fat	100 g	95	49	40	11
Chicken	white meat, without skin	100 g cooked	165	81	19	0
	with skin	100 g cooked	200	63	37	0
Egg		1 medium-sized	80	32	65	3
Frankfurter		1 medium-sized	170	16	82	2
Hamburger		100 g cooked	285	36	64	0
Kidney beans		100 g cooked	120	27	3	70
Lentils		100 g cooked	105	30	3	67
Milk	skimmed	10 cl	35	39	5	56
	whole	10 cl	65	21	49	30
Oats		250 g cooked	130	16	15	69
Peanut butter		2 tablespoons	190	16	71	13
Pizza	cheese	60 g slice	155	15	25	60
Plaice		100 g cooked	70	89	11	0
Potato	baked	1 medium-sized	215	8	1	91
Rice	brown	100 g cooked	115	8	5	87
Soya beans		100 g cooked	130	36	43	21
Spaghetti		100 g cooked	105	13	3	84
Tuna	in oil, drained	100 g	210	61	39	0
	in water, drained	100 g	110	94	6	0
Yogurt	plain, low-fat	100 g	60	33	22	45

The Facts about "Power Foods"

Among body builders and athletes, certain foods have acquired mythical reputations for building power and improving performance. As this chart illustrates, most of these foods contain no significant nutrients, and none of them has been shown to have any enhancing effect on athletic performance, appearance or health.

FOOD	CLAIM	COMMENT
B$_{15}$ (Pangamic acid)	Increases the delivery of oxygen to the cells and tissues	B$_{15}$ does not improve oxygen delivery. No evidence exists to show a vitamin function for this substance. Tablets from one manufacturer were found to contain only pure lactose (milk sugar).
Bee pollen	Enhances performance by increasing energy strength and stamina	Bee pollen does not possess any energy-producing substances and has failed to benefit exercisers. There is no research to support the claim that bee pollen enhances performance. Highly allergenic.
Bicarbonate of Soda	Increases muscle efficiency; enhances performance; helps reduce muscle fatigue by making blood more alkaline	Most studies, in which subjects have taken between 200 and 300 mg of bicarbonate of soda for every kilogram of body weight, have failed to link bicarbonate of soda with improved performance. Can cause diarrhoea
Brewer's yeast	Enhances performance	Although this product contains some B vitamins, it has not been shown to improve athletic performance or boost energy levels.
Caffeine	Supplies energy	Caffeine appears to have no beneficial effect on short-term, anaerobic exercise. Several studies contend that caffeine may improve performance in endurance activities requiring more than an hour of sustained effort. Negative effects include stomach upset, nervousness, increased water loss (due to diuretic properties), dizziness, nausea and headache.
Carnitine (Vitamin B-T)	Diminishes muscle fatigue and pain	No evidence has been found to support the claim. There is no dietary requirement for carnitine, so it is not considered a vitamin.
Gelatine	Boosts energy, improves endurance	Tests have failed to show any endurance benefit from gelatine or the amino acid glycine found in it.

FOOD	CLAIM	COMMENT
Ginseng root	Boosts energy and sustains endurance	No well-controlled studies have been conducted. Among the problems reported in ginseng users (especially those who have taken large amounts for long periods of time) are nervousness, insomnia, sore breasts, high blood pressure.
Kelp (Seaweed)	Increases energy, helps bones heal faster; a high-quality protein	Kelp has not been found to increase energy or aid in bone healing. Its protein is of poor quality and minimal. Dried kelp has been found to contain more than eight times as much iodine as iodized salt.
Liver	Increases endurance, builds strong muscles	Liver is high in iron and protein and is an extremely rich source of retinol, a form of vitamin A. However, liver should not be eaten daily, since a 100 g serving has 354 mg of cholesterol; 300 mg is the daily recommended limit. Liver also raises the concentration of purines (by-products of protein metabolism) in the blood, which may cause gout or kidney stones.
Raw eggs	High protein content builds muscle mass	Egg protein will not build muscle. Eggs are an excellent complete protein, but the yolk contains a great deal of cholesterol. **Do not eat raw eggs**; negative effects include nausea, appetite loss, and muscle pain and fatigue (cooked egg white has no harmful effects).
Wheat germ; Octacosanol (alcohol isolate extracted from wheat germ)	Improves performance, especially endurance; boosts energy	Wheat germ and octacosanol have no known energy-producing effects.

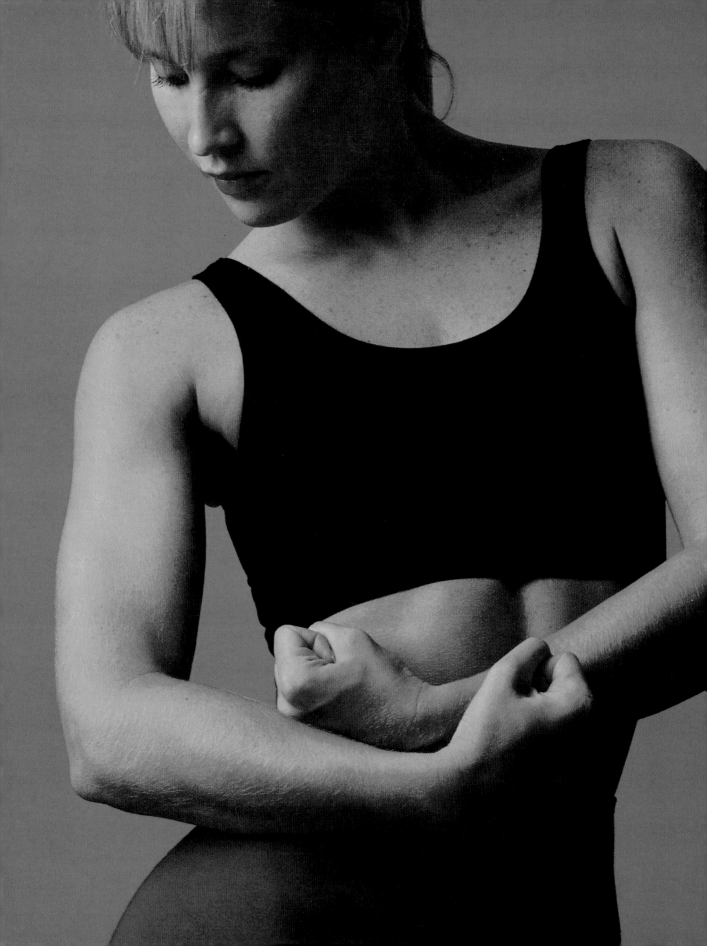

CHAPTER TWO

Advanced Shaping and Toning

Tough versions of push-ups, sit-ups and other muscle-building callisthenics

The exercises in this chapter provide a workout that focuses on shaping and toning all of the major muscle groups. Many of the exercises are based on classic callisthenics movements, such as push-ups and sit-ups, but the versions shown here place more of a demand on your muscles and also target them from different angles to enhance their definition. These movements are also excellent for building muscular endurance: one study showed that endurance improved in subjects at the rate of 10 per cent per week when they performed 15 to 25 repetitions of an exercise over a period of seven weeks.

The key to getting the most from a callisthenics workout is variety: firming even one set of muscles requires more than one movement because most exercises not only work specific muscles, but focus on certain portions of a muscle. For example, when you do a traditional sit-up, you are mostly working the upper portion of your abdomen. Your oblique muscles, which taper to define your waist, are hardly exercised at all. By performing the exercises on pages 28-37, you will rotate your torso to work these muscles.

You do not need weights or other elaborate equipment to perform these exercises. A few of them require one or two chairs, but most rely solely on the positioning of your limbs and torso to supply the resistance. The fact that they do not involve weights does not mean that these exercises are easy: you need to be in fair condition to perform them properly (see the self-assessment tests on pages 12-13). Even if you are in good shape, you should begin slowly, performing each exercise with the number of repetitions that places a demand on your muscles without straining them.

Because your muscles need time to recover, it is a good idea to alternate exercises for different parts of your body on different days. You will find that your workout capacity will grow faster than if you exercise the same muscles every day, since toning and growth take place during recuperation after you have stressed the muscle. The box on the opposite page provides guidelines for using these exercises in a progressive-training programme that strengthens muscles by gradually increasing the amount of work they must do.

Using your body weight for resistance requires that you be especially careful to use proper form. For example, it is easy to bend at the waist when doing a push-up, but you will work harder and get more from the exercise if you keep your body aligned correctly and your arms placed properly. For this reason, it is better to do 20 perfect push-ups than 50 push-ups in bad form.

If you cannot complete the suggested number of repetitions (reps), do them in sets. For example, if 20 reps of a negative sit-up are prescribed, perform two sets of 10 or four sets of five with short breaks of 10 to 15 seconds between the sets until you can manage to do all the reps with no break. Perform the exercises as fast as you can while still maintaining the proper form. You will build more endurance by doing fewer repetitions in quick succession than by doing the full amount slowly.

Pay close attention to your breathing while you perform the exercises. The proper way to breathe is to exhale during the exertion phase of an exercise and inhale during the relaxation phase. Many people unconsciously begin to hold their breath, especially towards the end of a series of repetitions. Researchers have theorized that doing so — in effect, pushing the inhaled air against your chest and throat — may give the illusion of assisting the chest muscles. By pressing on your heart and forcing it to empty blood into the arteries rapidly, the compressed air in your lungs makes your blood pressure rise abruptly. The air also presses on the relatively thin-walled veins leading to the heart, making the return of blood into the heart much slower and causing an abrupt drop in blood pressure. You can become dizzy, see "spots" or even faint. Also, because the heart works hard to pump blood to the muscles when you exercise, it needs more oxygen

Workout Progressions

◆ If you are not already exercising on a regular schedule, begin by working out three times a week. Do as many repetitions for each exercise as you find comfortable, and then an additional rep for each exercise if possible.

◆ You can train progressively by adding more repetitions to each set of exercises you do. Then increase the total number of sets you perform. Finally, add to the number of days per week that you work out. Do not increase too quickly or you may be injured.

◆ Steadily increasing the number of repetitions and/or sets you perform is an effective way to develop, but it can be boring. An alternative is to train progressively with a sequential plan:

- **Week One:** Perform the number of sets you can do comfortably for each area of the body in each of your three workout sessions.

- **Week Two:** Add repetitions in increments of five to each set of exercises.

- **Week Three:** Add repetitions in increments of five to each set.

- **Week Four:** Add an additional set with the original number of reps for each exercise.

- **Week Five:** Repeat Week Two.
- **Week Six:** Repeat Week Three.
- **Week Seven:** Repeat Week Four.
- **Week Eight:** Repeat Week Three.
- **Week Nine:** Repeat Week Four.

◆ By this time, your training session should take at least 30 minutes. To increase further, add another workout to your training week.

itself. Restricted blood flow means less oxygen for the heart rather than more. In addition, holding your breath during exercise increases intra-abdominal pressure and may even cause a hernia.

Along with breathing steadily and deliberately, it is important to warm up properly before you begin your workout. Warming up increases blood flow to the muscles and the temperature in the muscle core. As a result, your muscles should be able to work faster and more efficiently, and their ability to use oxygen should improve. In addition, warming up should make the blood vessels in the muscles dilate, increasing blood flow to the area, so that oxygen reaches muscle tissue faster and waste products are removed more quickly as well.

Cooling down after exercise is also necessary to remove waste products that accumulate in the muscles as a result of exertion. Stopping exercise abruptly can cause a sudden drop in blood pressure because, when the heart stops pumping hard, the blood can pool in the veins. Good warm-ups and cool-downs are repetitive and aerobic, like running on the spot, at a moderate level of exertion.

If possible, perform your exercises in front of a full-length mirror, and pay close attention to the line your torso makes and the angle of your legs in the various exercises. Wear tights, a leotard or shorts so that your clothing does not obscure your image.

The Upper Body

The muscles that can be developed to contribute the most definition to your physique are those of the upper torso and arms — pectorals, deltoids, latissimus dorsi across the middle back and the smaller muscles of the back, biceps and triceps. The fact that these muscles are, in many people, the least exercised body parts means that they often respond quickly to training. Since the upper body generally stores less fat than other body areas, the definition that occurs is more readily apparent.

In the push-ups, hip rotation, hip drop and the scapular shrug, shown on these two and the following four pages, you use your body weight for resistance. The principle to remember when you perform all these exercises is to keep your torso in one plane; do not bend forwards at the hip or arch your back.

Focus your gaze at a particular place at about eye level a metre or so away in order to keep your head level while performing the exercises. This will help you to concentrate on your motion as well. It is important to continue breathing normally as you work out. Perform 15 to 20 repetitions of each exercise.

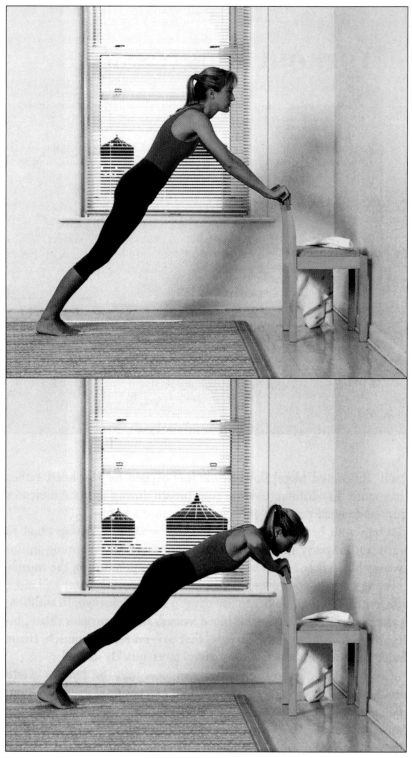

Support your aligned body at a 45-degree angle to the floor by holding the back of a chair or other stable piece of furniture *(top)*. Without bending at the waist, lower yourself towards the chair *(above)*. Return to the starting position.

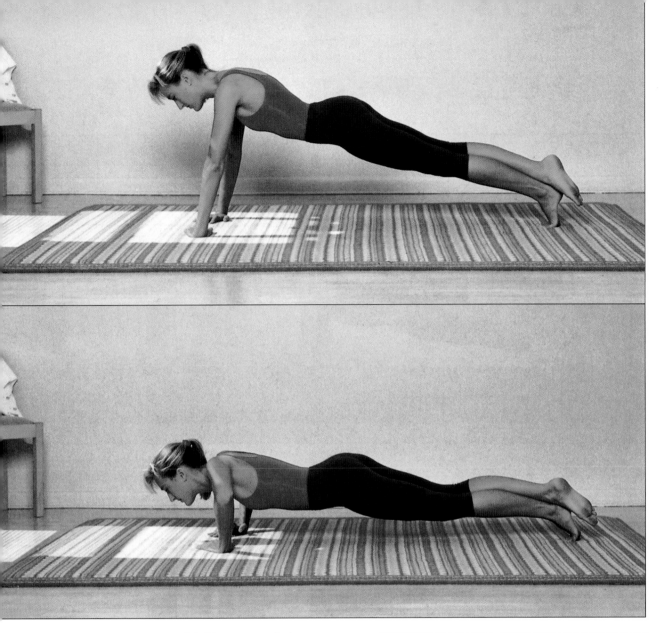

To work your deltoids, cross one foot over the other and support your weight with your hands pointed inwards *(top)*. Use your abdominal muscles to keep your body rigid as you lower yourself towards the floor *(above)*. If the classic push-up is too difficult, perform the knee push-up *(right)*, making certain to keep your body aligned as you lower and raise yourself.

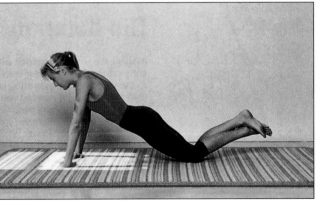

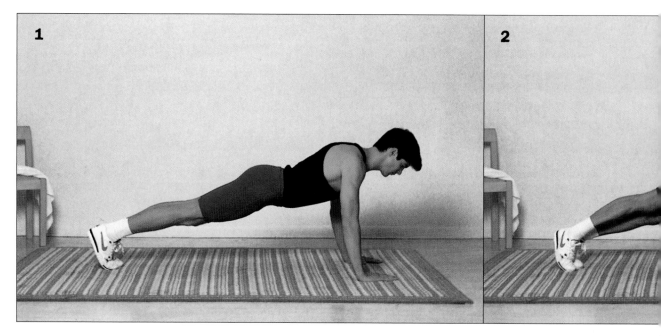

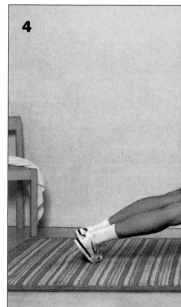

Hip Rotation

Assume the push-up position with your feet together and your arms extended at shoulder level (1). Keeping your body rigid, rotate your right hip outwards, lifting yourself up on to the fingers of your right hand as you turn (2). Lower yourself to the floor as if for a standard push-up (3). Then raise yourself and rotate your left hip outwards, lifting yourself on to the fingers of your left hand (4). Lower yourself to the floor again (5).

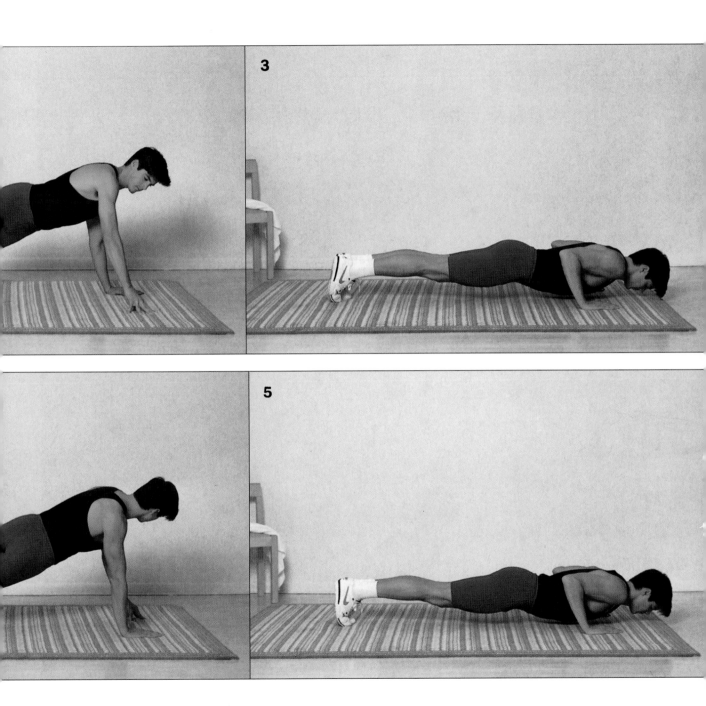

Hip Drop

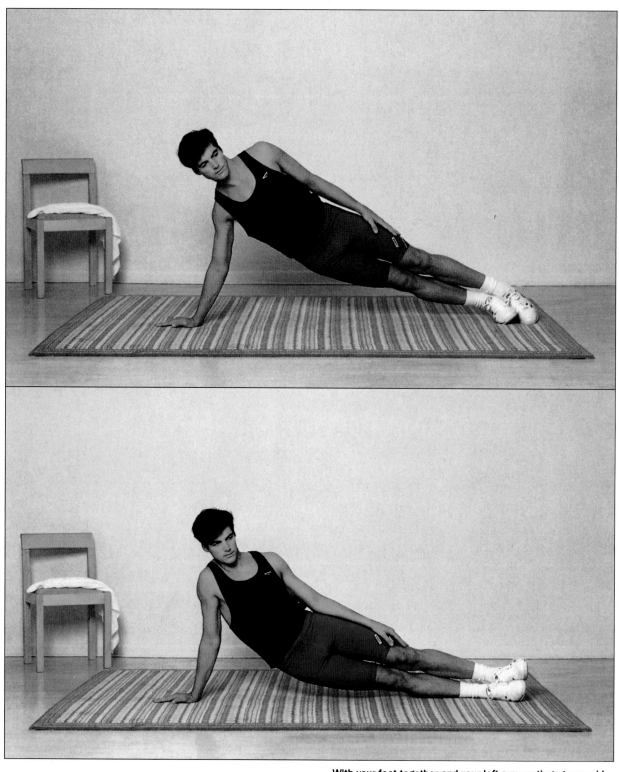

With your feet together and your left arm resting at your side, support your aligned body on your extended right arm *(top)*. Bend at the waist to allow your right hip to drop towards the floor *(above)*. Raise yourself again to the starting position.

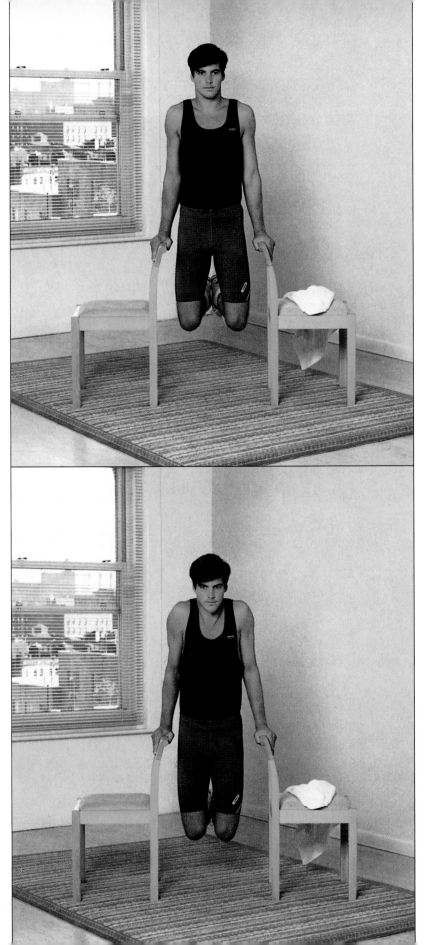

Scapular Shrug

Support yourself between two stable chairs and bend your knees so that your lower legs are parallel to the floor *(left)*. Then hunch your shoulders, allowing your body to drop lower between the chairs *(below)*. Return to the starting position.

27

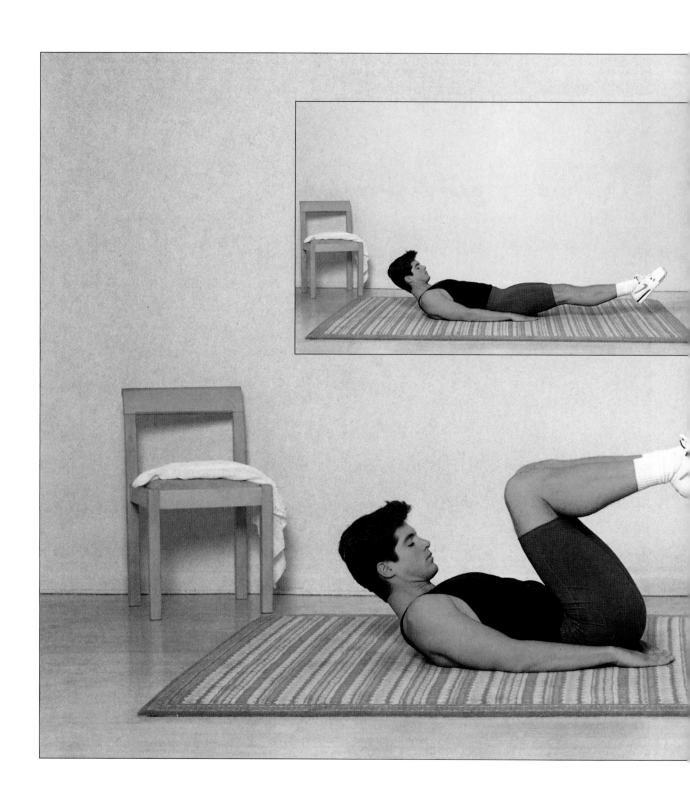

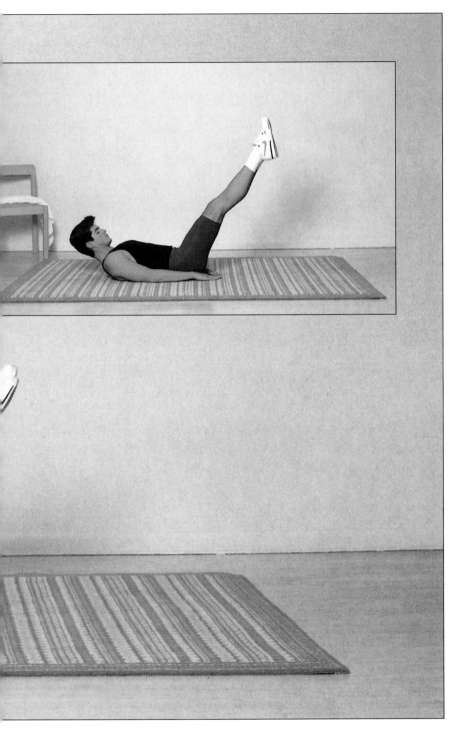

The Middle Body

The paramount sign of looking truly fit is an abdomen that is visibly well toned. The big muscle of the middle body, the rectus abdominis, which stretches from the breastbone to the pelvis, is divided by tendinous bands that hold it in place. These bands are responsible for the sectional appearance of toned abdominals. But you must be quite trim for these muscle divisions to be visible.

Straight-leg sit-ups are no longer the exercise of choice for the abdominals. Instead leg extensions, curls and bent-leg sit-ups are recommended because, while they are demanding enough to work even well-developed muscles, they are safe for the lower back. However, if you have a history of lower back pain you should avoid all such exercises, including the ones that are shown in this section.

When you perform the exercises shown on these and the following eight pages, pay special attention to your breathing. Exhale during the most difficult part; inhale during the easy portion. Perform 15 to 20 repetitions for each exercise.

DOUBLE LEG LIFT Lie on the floor with the small of your back pressed to the mat, your hands under your buttocks and your head at a 45-degree angle to the floor. Lift your legs off the mat slightly *(left inset)*. Raise your legs high, keeping your knees straight but not locked *(right inset)*. Then bend your knees towards your head *(left)*. Return to the starting position. Avoid this exercise if you suffer from lower back pain.

Double Leg Extension

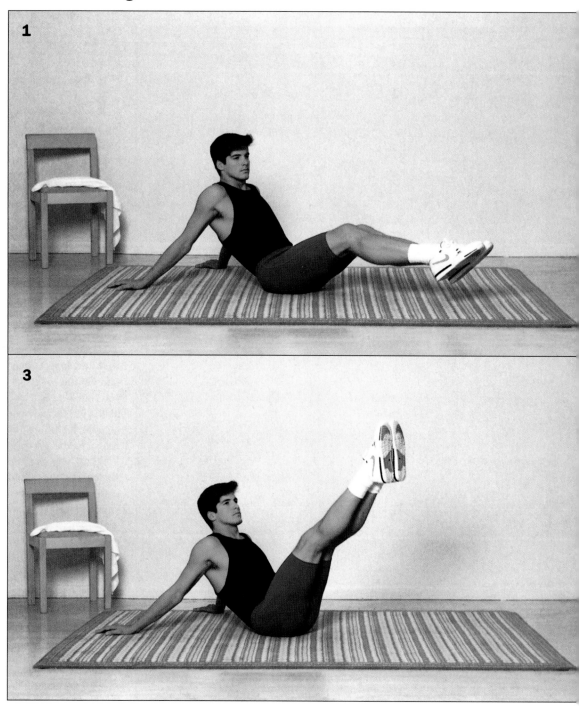

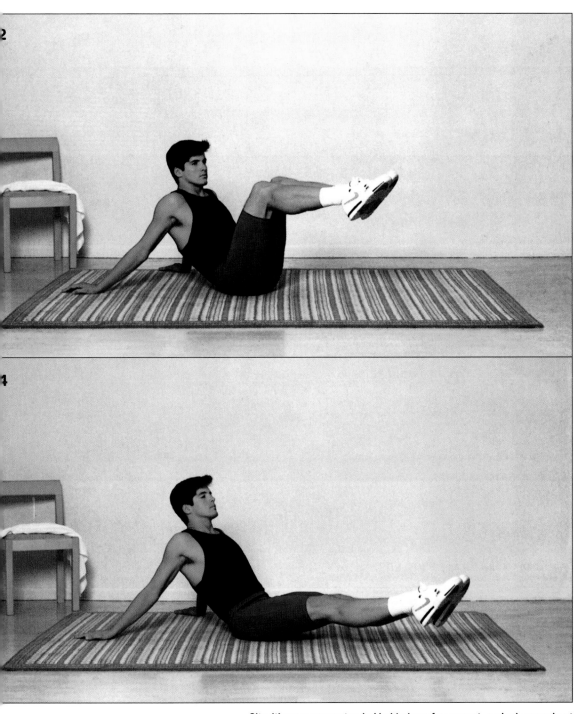

Sit with your arms extended behind you for support, and raise your bent legs off the floor with your feet together (1). Bend your knees and draw them towards your chest (2). Then lift and extend your legs, pointing your toes towards the ceiling (3). Lower your legs almost to the floor, keeping your knees extended but not locked (4). Avoid this exercise if you suffer from lower back pain.

Double Leg Raise

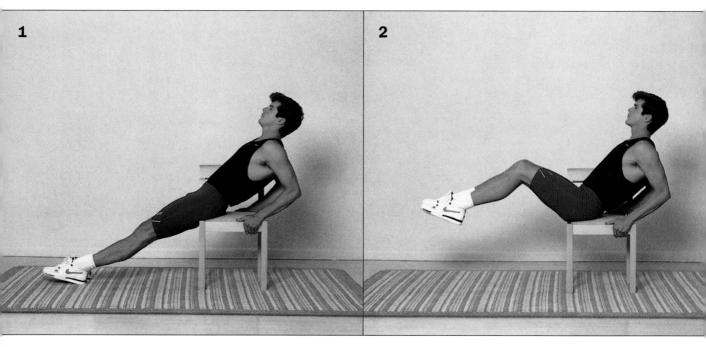

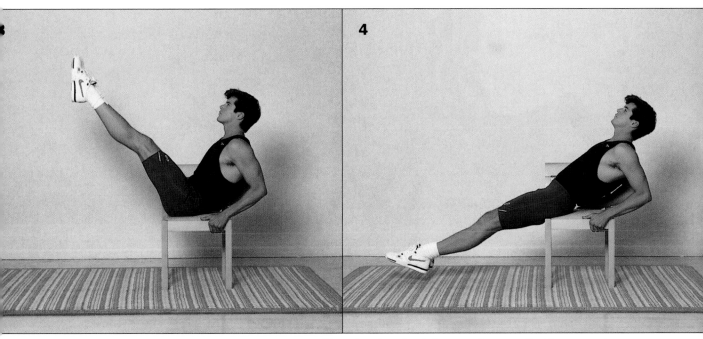

Sit on the edge of a chair, supporting yourself with your arms bent behind you and holding on to the seat. Extend your legs so that your body is at a 45-degree angle to the floor (1). Bend your knees and lift your feet to the height of the seat (2). Then extend your legs and raise them as high as you can (3). Keeping your knees extended, lower your legs to the floor (4). Avoid this exercise if you suffer from lower back pain.

Negative Sit-Up

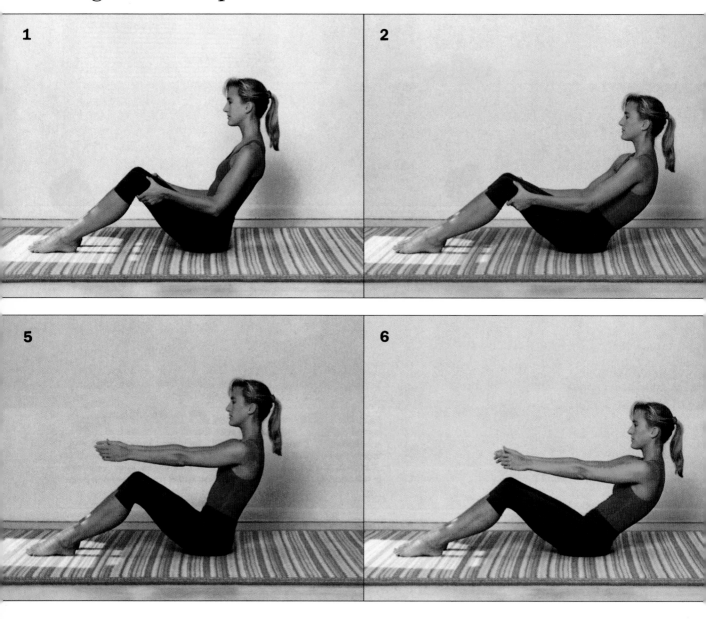

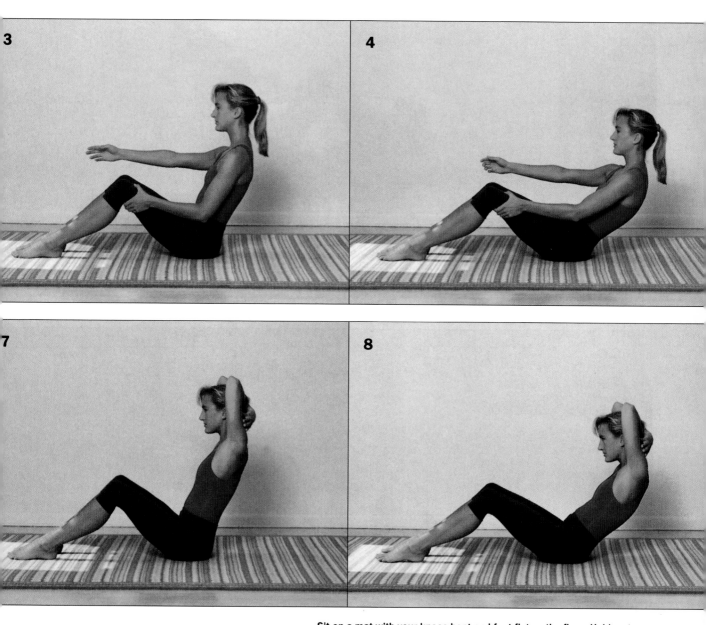

Sit on a mat with your knees bent and feet flat on the floor. Hold on to your thighs close to your knees (1). Round your back as you lower yourself towards the floor to the point where your arms are almost extended (2). Return to the starting position, and reach forwards with your right arm (3). Keeping your arm extended, round your back as you lower yourself again, holding your left thigh firmly (4). Repeat steps 3 and 4 with your left arm. Then reach forwards with both arms (5), and lower yourself, rounding your back (6). Repeat the sequence with your arms crossed behind your head as shown (7, 8). Avoid this exercise if you suffer from lower back pain.

Total Body Curl

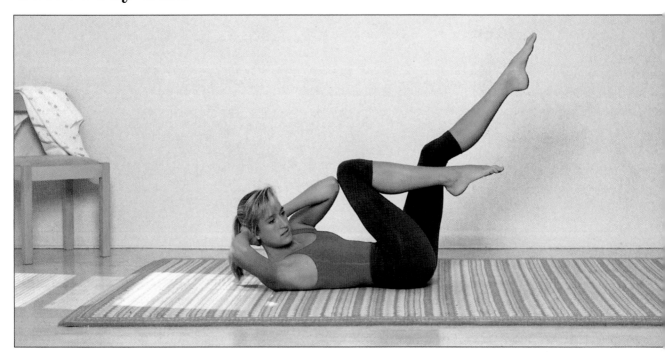

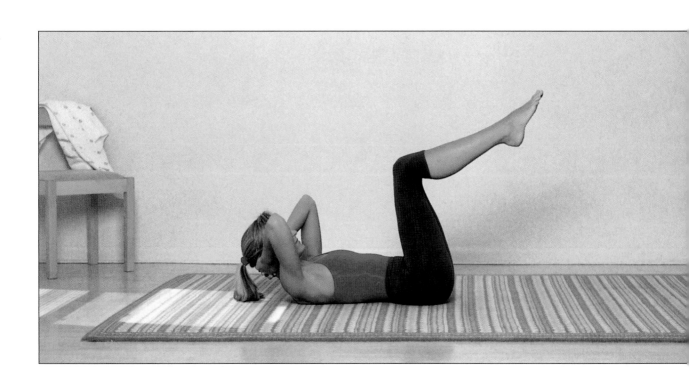

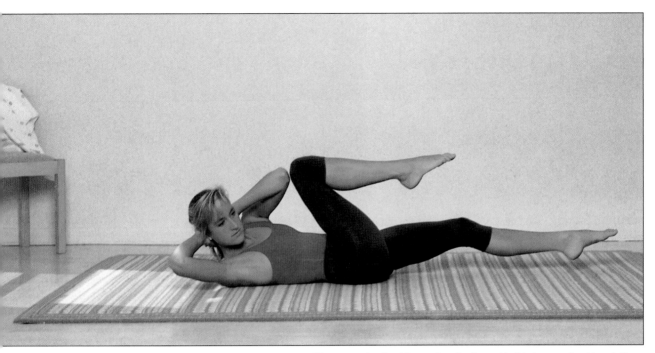

Lie on your back with your hands clasped behind your raised head. Draw your right knee towards your left elbow and raise your left leg as high as you can, keeping your knee bent slightly *(above, opposite)*. Lower your left leg towards the floor, straightening your knee *(above)*.

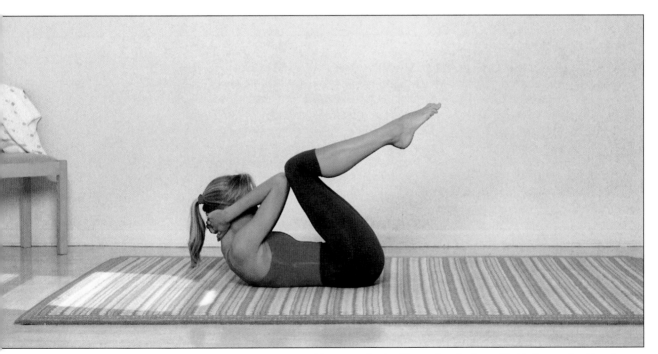

Lie on your back with your hands clasped behind your raised head, your thighs perpendicular to your torso and your knees bent *(opposite)*. Draw your knees to your elbows, keeping your toes pointed *(above)*. Make sure the small of your back is pressed against the mat. Avoid this exercise if you suffer from lower back pain.

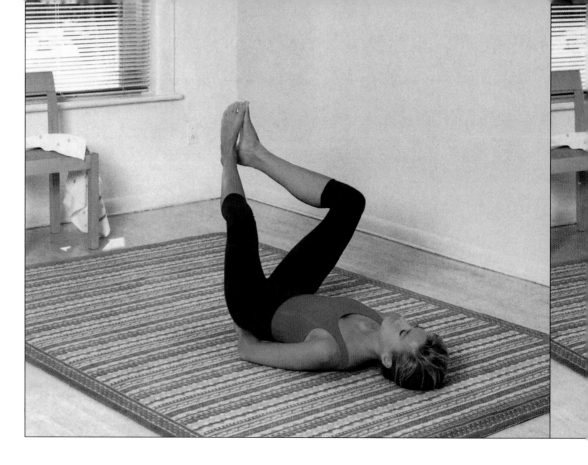

The Lower Body

Any exercises for toning the muscles of the lower body have to be particularly demanding, since these muscles are often the strongest. Still, toning them is important, especially the muscles that form the buttocks and those of the inner thigh, since neither of these groups is adequately exercised by everyday activities such as walking and carrying shopping.

The exercises that appear on this page and the following five pages are unusual because, if you do them incorrectly, you will find them much too easy. In order to do them correctly, you must supply resistance by tensing your muscles in isometric contraction while you perform the movement of the exercises.

The exercises on pages 44-47 are especially difficult since they tax the muscles of your back as well as your hamstrings, quadriceps and adductors of your thighs. If you are prone to lower back pain, avoid these exercises. To strengthen your thighs and buttocks without stressing your lower back, you should perform the hamstring-gluteus bend on page 48.

The squats and demi-squats on pages 50-53 develop the quadriceps along with the gluteals. Be sure to exhale during the exertion phase of the exercise and inhale during the relaxation phase.

Perform the same exercises on both sides of your body, alternating with each repetition for a total of 15 to 20 reps on each side.

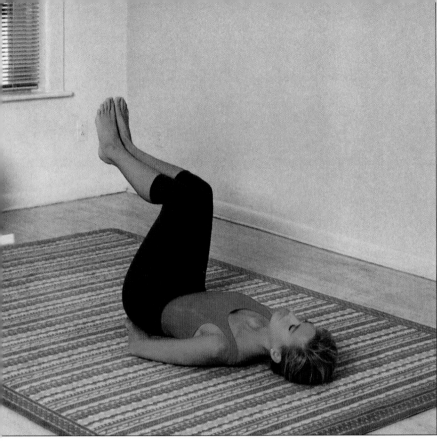

TRIANGLE PRESS Lie on your back with your hands placed under your buttocks, your feet together and your knees apart *(opposite)*. As you tense the muscles of your inner thighs, press your knees together forcibly *(left)*.

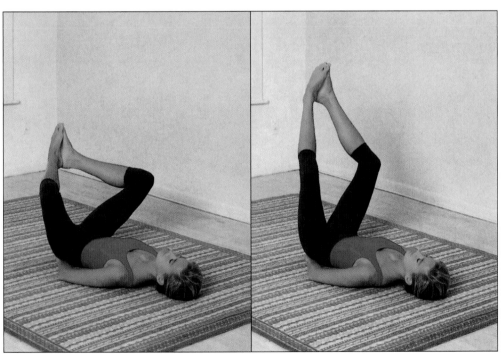

TRIANGLE LIFT Lie on your back with your feet together, your knees apart and your hands placed under your buttocks *(above, left)*. Tense the muscles of your inner thighs as you press your feet towards the ceiling forcibly *(above)*. Return to the starting position.

Inner Thigh Lift

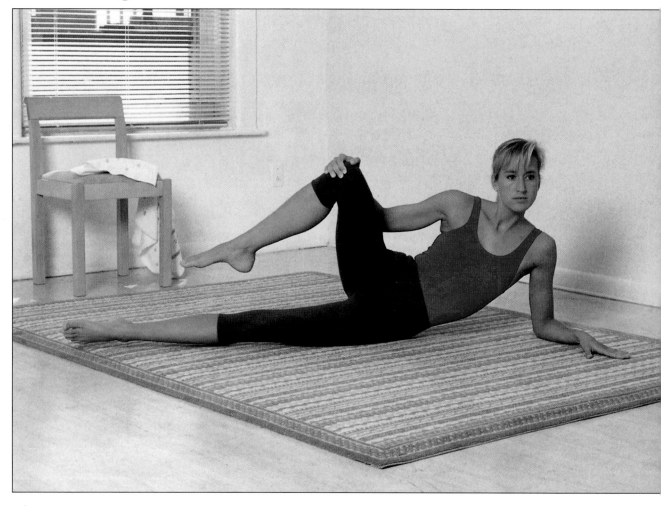

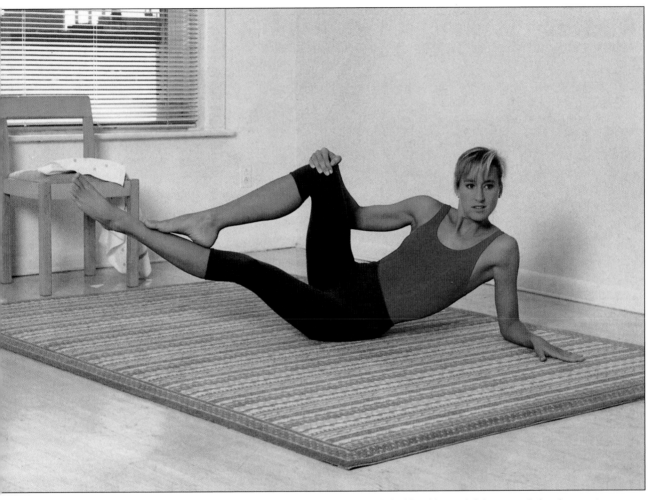

Lie on your left side with your left leg extended and support yourself on your left arm. Hold your bent right knee with your right hand *(opposite)*. Without rotating backwards, raise your extended left leg to touch your right foot *(above)*. Return to the starting position.

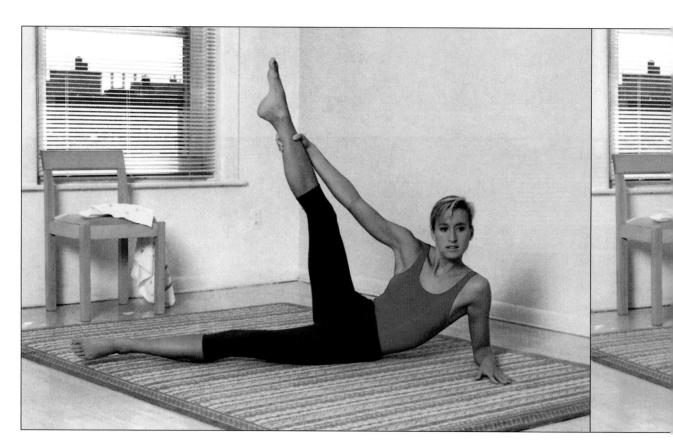

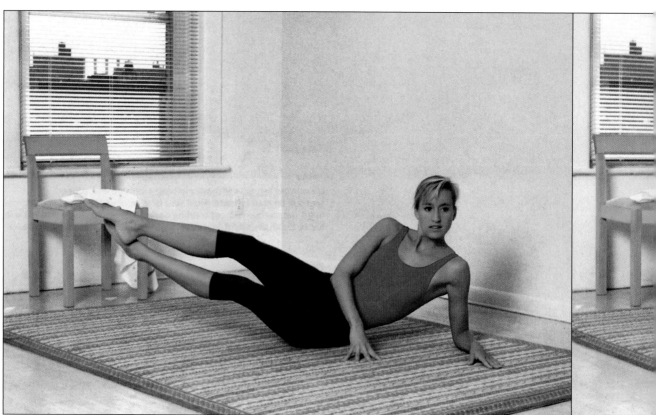

Hip Balance

Lie on your left side with your left leg extended and hold your raised right leg with your right hand *(opposite)*. Lift your extended left leg towards your right leg *(left)*. Return to the starting position.

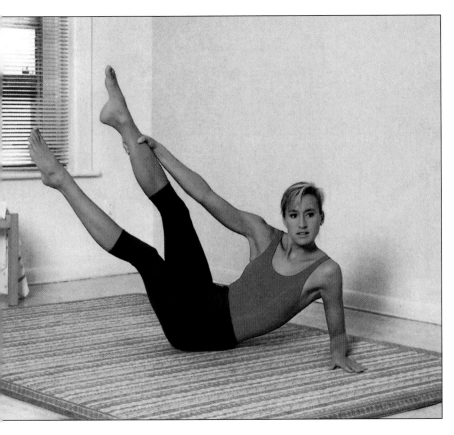

Diagonal Thigh Lift

Support yourself on your left side with your bent left arm and use your right arm to brace yourself. Raise your extended legs — crossed at the ankles — about 30 centimetres off the floor *(opposite)*. Then raise both legs as high as you can without losing your balance *(left)*. Return to the starting position.

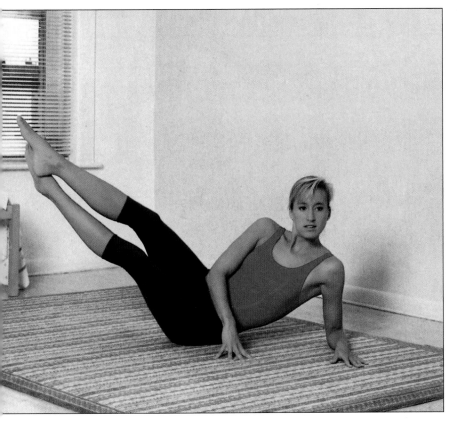

43

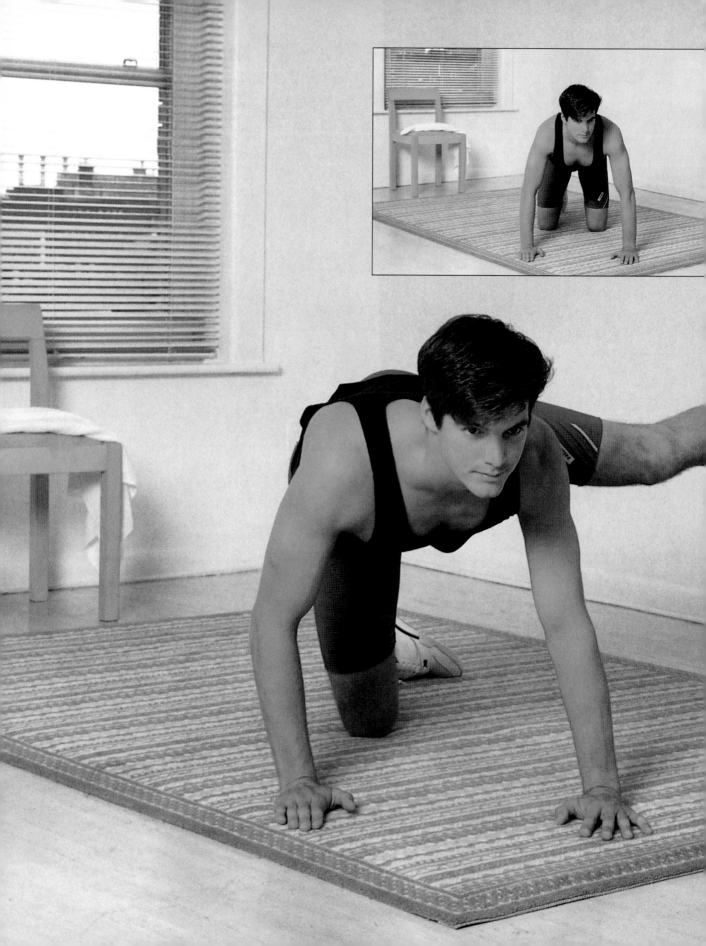

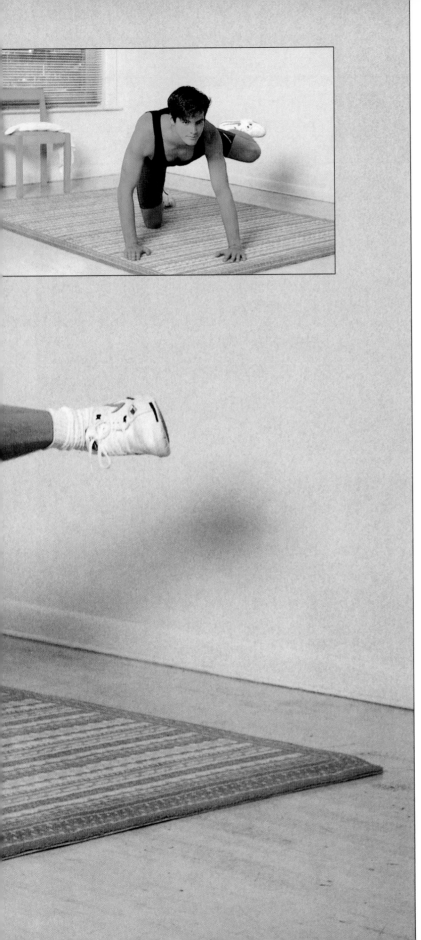

Outer Thigh Lift/1

Position yourself on your knees on a mat with your hands placed shoulder-width apart *(left inset)*. Raise your left leg out to the side, keeping your knee bent and your foot parallel to the floor, as high as possible *(right inset)*. Then straighten your knee by bringing your foot forwards, so that your extended leg is perpendicular to your torso *(left)*. Return to the starting position.

Outer Thigh Lift/2

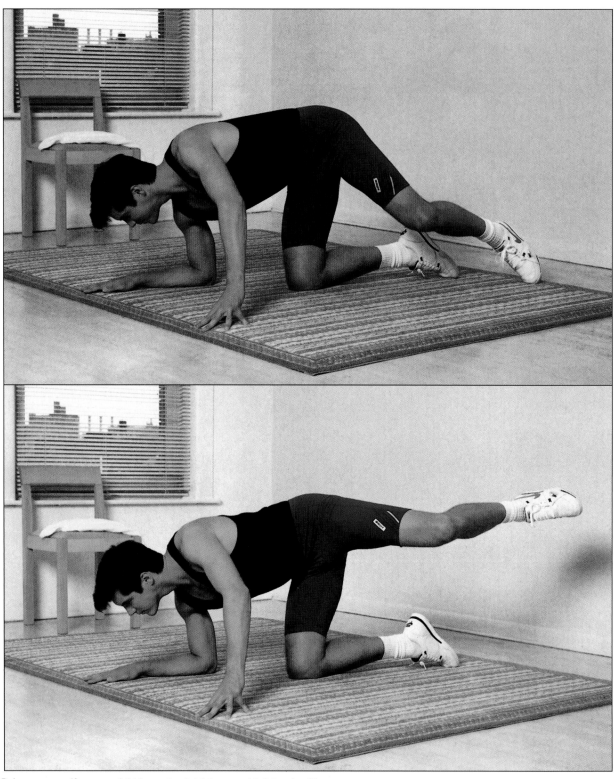

Balance yourself on your right knee, bent right arm and left hand, with your left leg extended behind you *(top)*. Raise your left leg out to the side and behind you *(above)*. Return to the starting position.

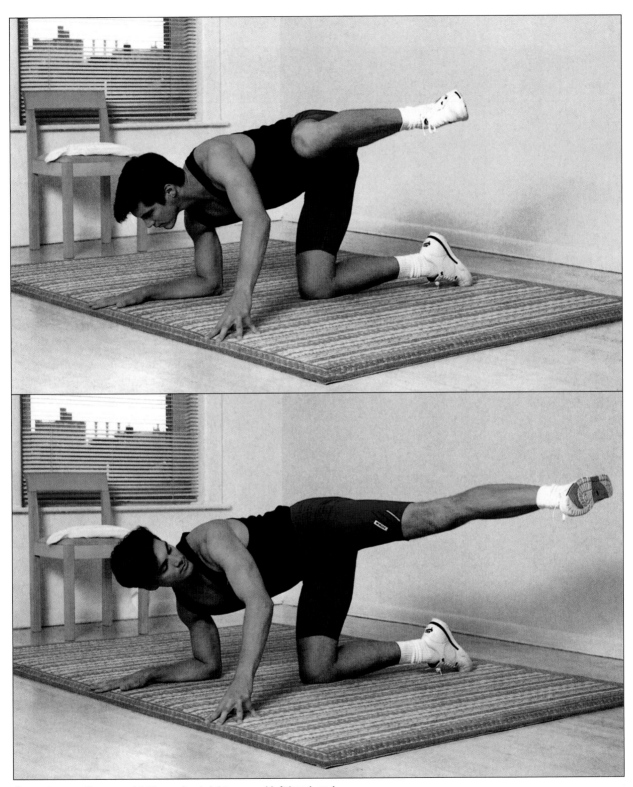

Support yourself on your right knee, bent right arm and left hand, and raise your bent left leg out to the side *(top)*. Look at your leg as you extend it and flex your foot *(above)*. Return to the starting position.

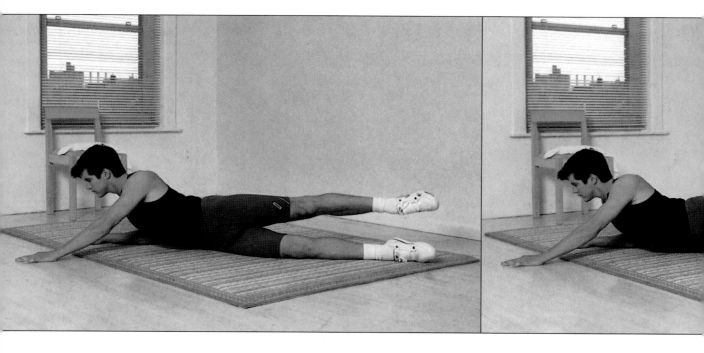

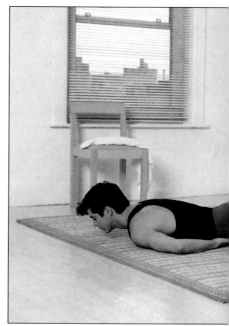

Hamstring-Gluteus Bend

Lie on your stomach with your hands under your hips, your head resting on your chin and your left leg bent so that your foot is parallel to the floor *(right)*. Raise your left leg off the floor, keeping your knee bent *(far right)*. Return to the starting position.

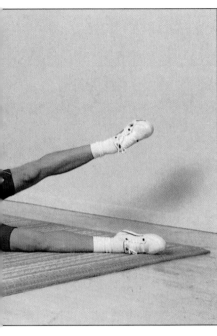

Hamstring Lift

Lie on the floor on your right side, supporting yourself on your bent right arm, and assisting your balance with your extended left arm. Hold your extended left leg about 15 centimetres from your extended right leg *(far left)*.
Raise your left leg as high as you can *(left)*. Return to the starting position.

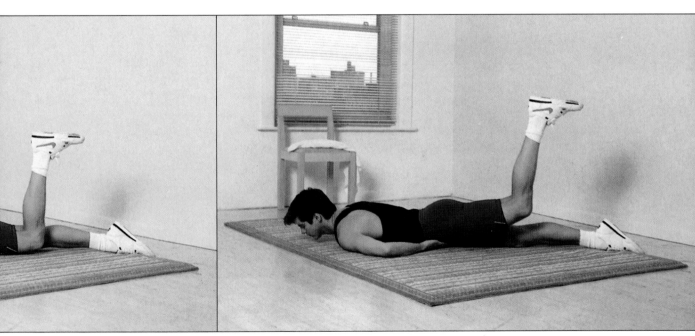

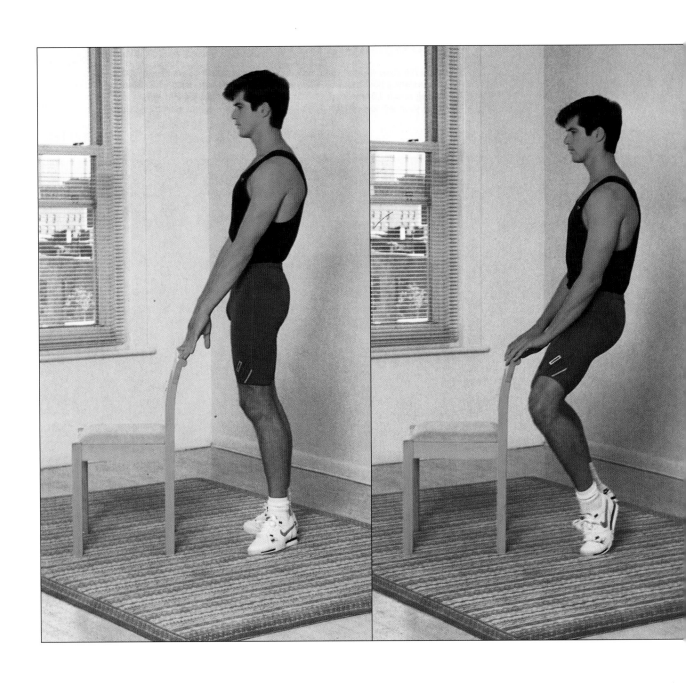

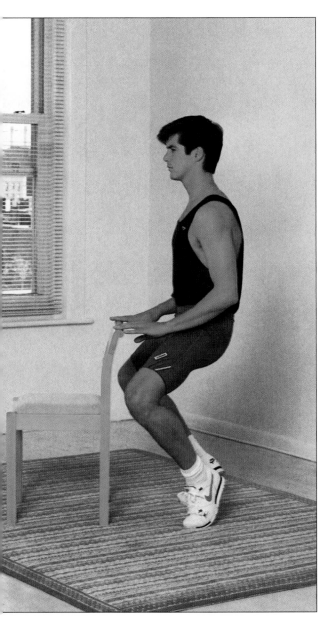

Demi-Squat

Stand with your feet comfortably apart and your pelvis tucked, facing a chair or other stable piece of furniture with your hands resting on its back *(far left)*. Using the chair to balance, bend your knees outwards and rise up on your toes *(centre)*. Lower yourself until your forearms are parallel to the floor, keeping your pelvis tucked *(left)*. Return to the starting position.

Squat

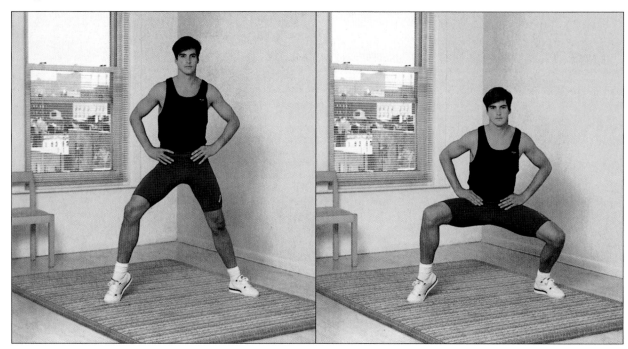

With your hands on your hips and your feet spread apart, stand on your left foot and your right toes *(above, left)*. Squat by bending your knees until your thighs are parallel to the floor *(above)*, then stand.

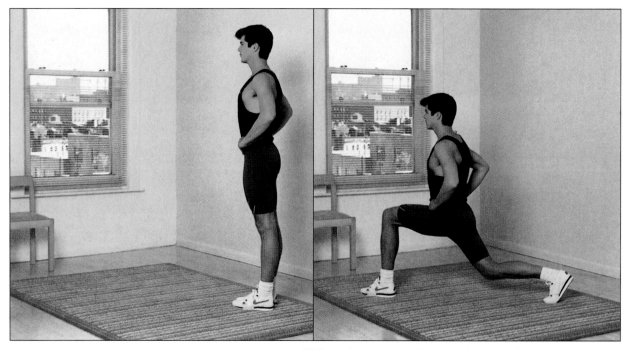

With your hands on your hips, stand with your feet comfortably apart *(above, left)*. Squat by lunging forwards on your left foot, bending your right knee to the floor *(above)*; then stand erect.

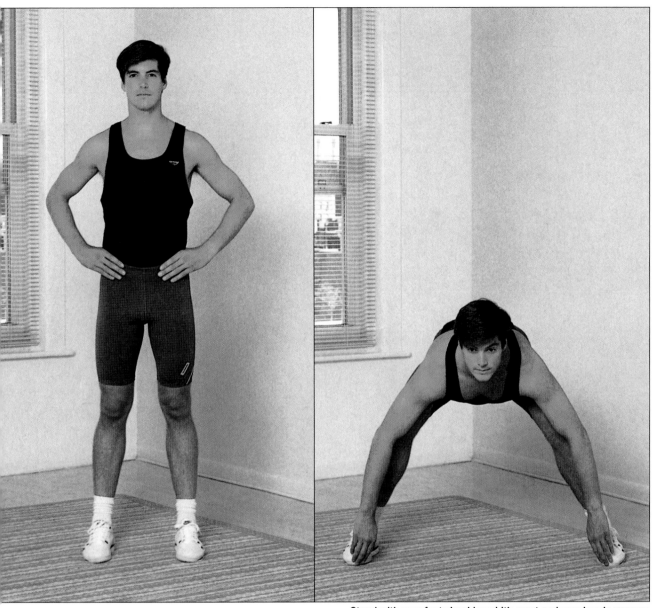

Stand with your feet shoulder-width apart and your hands on your hips *(above, left)*. Squat by moving your right leg to the side and bending at the waist and knees. Touch your feet with your hands *(above)*. Return to the starting position.

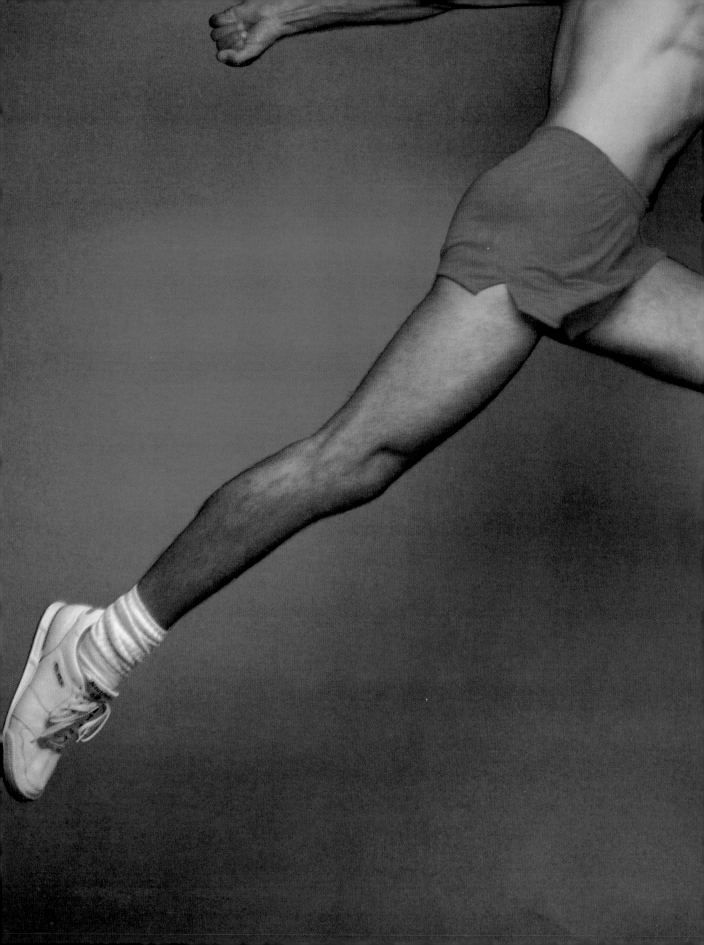

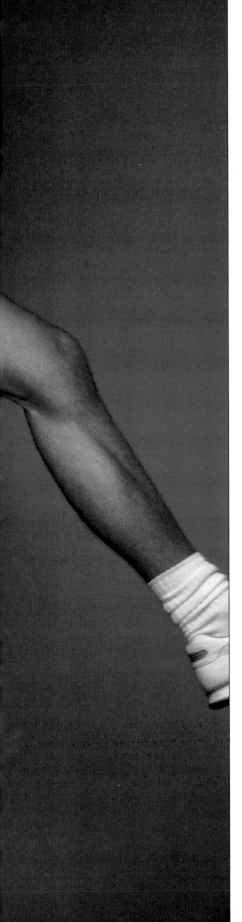

CHAPTER THREE

Plyometrics

*Leaping, bounding and throwing
for explosive bursts of power*

What if you could utilize a special reflex to build momentum rather than lose it when you jump, leap or catch and then throw a ball? Or if you could actually increase your power by changing direction when you run or jump? Athletes in Eastern Europe and the Soviet Union discovered a way to do this in the mid-1960s, using an exercise called plyometrics. The power created by plyometrics is usually characterized as "explosive", because it concentrates a large amount of force in a very short period of time. Now Western athletes — soccer, rugby, basketball and tennis players — are among those who find this training effective, especially in sports that require quick acceleration.

The basis for plyometric exercise is the fact that muscles and tendons are elastic, and so can recoil when stretched. The primary objective of plyometrics is to convert this recoil energy during a muscular contraction into an equal and opposite force. The training that is required to accomplish this involves the rapid stretching of a muscle to produce a forceful movement in a short period of time. This occurs, for example, when you cock your arm to throw a ball, or squat quickly before performing a vertical jump.

Although each sport requires a different style of plyometric training, depending on the muscles used for the particular activity, the various plyometric movements all utilize three distinct phases: a vigorous stretch, a transition period and a final reaction and motion.

During the first phase, these exercises rapidly stretch the muscles that are involved. This stretching can occur in the muscles of your legs, for instance, as you land from a jump on the spot, or you can experience it in the muscles of your arms and shoulders as you get ready to throw a weighted medicine ball.

This first step usually produces a "cocking motion", because your muscles act like coiled springs that store potential energy as they elongate. The crouch you assume just before you jump for a rebound while playing basketball is another example of this action. As you crouch, the muscles in your legs stretch and set in motion a muscular reflex known as the myotatic reflex — a stretch reflex of the muscle spindle. This reflex, which takes place during the first phase of all plyometric activity, activates a powerful neuromuscular stimulus from the spinal cord to the muscles that consequently helps them contract more forcefully than they would without the preparatory cocking motion. That is why the crouch before jumping for a basketball rebound results in a higher leap than merely standing with your hands in the air before grabbing the ball.

The second phase of a plyometric exercise is the transition between the initial eccentric contraction and the final reaction. Exercise physiologists who have studied plyometrics call this transition the amortization phase. Successful plyometric training focuses on making the amortization phase as a brief as possible.

The final phase is the concentric contraction of your muscles, when they tighten and grow shorter. This should take place as quickly as possible, so that the resulting motion is a rapid "explosion" of force.

Because of the swift and intense concentration of force during plyometrics, these exercises should be performed sparingly and with caution. They are not for beginner exercisers or people who are not at least moderately physically fit. You should fully master the simpler exercises before attempting the more difficult manoeuvres. The plyometric exercises shown in this chapter are arranged in order of increasing difficulty for each area of the body.

The more elementary plyometrics *(see pages 59-61)* are the safest and also require the least equipment. These exercises should be performed once or twice a week for four to six weeks before you progress to the more stressful exercises. In particular, strenuous activities, such as in-depth jumps *(see pages 80-82)*, which introduce powerful forces on your knees and tendons, should only be performed if you are able to do a squat with one and a half times your body weight on a barbell

Equipment for Plyometrics

◆ For running and jumping exercises, you will need a resilient surface at least 25 metres long, such as a wooden gym floor, with adequate space for bounding and leaping. For some exercises, working outdoors on grass is best, either in a large back garden or on a playing field.

◆ To work out indoors, you will need a sizable exercise mat that is dense enough to make jumping safe and comfortable and that will not slide when you land on it.

◆ The plyometrics exercises on pages 78-83 require the use of a raised jumping surface. You can use either a step, a bench or a box made of wood and covered with a mat or padding that you can make or buy. Depending on your height and your jumping ability, this box should measure 20, 30 or 45 centimetres on each side for beginners, and it should be sturdy enough to support three times your body weight. You may want to use a 60-centimetre box for more advanced training.

◆ For the cone hops on pages 70-73, you will need 15-centimetre plastic cones similar to those used as lane markers on motorways. You can find them in sports-equipment shops but you could substitute soft household objects of similar height instead. These should be sturdy and stable, but soft enough not to cause injury if you fall on them.

◆ A medicine ball is used for the plyometrics movements on pages 84-89. These dense balls were previously made only of leather in the size of a basketball, but now they come in various sizes, and range in weight from 1.5 to 7 kilograms. They are usually covered with leather or polyurethane. You can find them in sports-equipment shops.

across your shoulders, or if you have prepared for these exercises with the previous plyometrics demonstrated in this chapter.

Exercises that require explosive force can injure you if you do not warm up sufficiently. An aerobic warm-up such as jogging for five to 10 minutes or cycling on a stationary bicycle should bring the core of your muscles to a safe temperature, and increase the blood supply to your peripheral tissues adequately. And, of course, after your plyometrics workout, you should also take five to 10 minutes to cool down, by performing simple stretches, without bouncing, or a slow aerobic routine similar to a warm-up.

If you train by yourself, without the benefit of a coach or trainer, you should never do plyometrics more than once a week. Do not perform them with ankle, wrist or chest weights, because they increase the chance of injury while decreasing the benefit of the exercise by slowing your reaction time.

For best results, plyometrics should be supplemented with sprint training and weightlifting. Children should not perform advanced plyometrics because they are too stressful for their joints; on their own, though, youngsters often take part in activities such as skipping, bounding and jumping, which are the exercises you should include at the start of your plyometrics programme.

The Lower Body

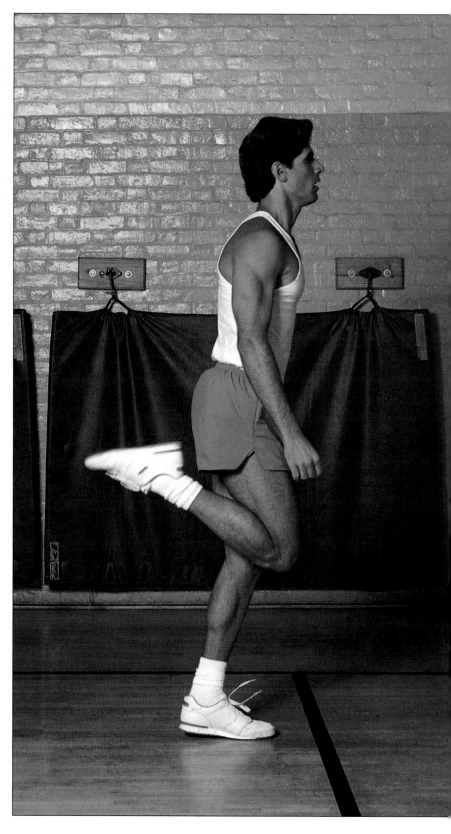

Lower body plyometrics are exercises that develop the legs primarily but, like all plyometric exercises, they require the effort of your upper body as well.

Once you have warmed up sufficiently, perform the exercises in the order given, beginning with the jumps on the spot, then the standing jumps, multiple hops and bounding. The plyometrics begin in earnest with the cone hops, since these are the first exercises in the sequence that require you to land and then take off again immediately.

Your warm-ups can include running on the spot, as shown here, or the hip kicker (see page 59) and the split squat walk (see page 60). Always stretch before and after your warm-ups to loosen your muscles.

To perform the cone hops on pages 70-73, you will require 15-centimetre cones made of plastic or rubber that are available in sports-equipment shops. Use three cones to begin with, and work your way up to five. You may substitute stuffed toys, or other soft household objects, so long as they are stable and have the necessary height. Be sure not to choose an object you could hurt yourself with should you land on it.

First perform the lead-up exercises shown on pages 58-61, which you can use as warm-ups. Then, for the exercises that follow, begin by performing three sets of five repetitions and work up to three sets of 10 reps. The harder the exercise, the fewer reps you should do initially.

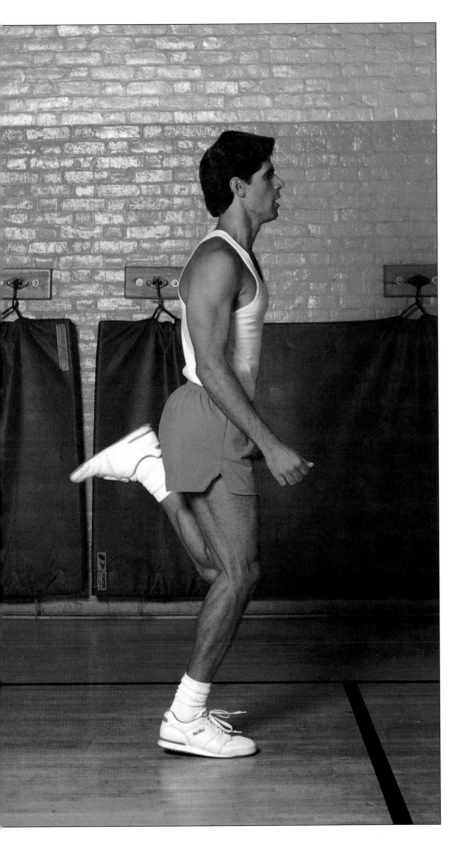

HIP KICKER Stand with your arms at your sides and your feet shoulder-width apart. Lean forwards slightly with your back straight. Run on the spot, keeping your knees pointed straight down. Try to kick your right buttock with your right heel *(opposite)*, then your left buttock with your left heel *(left)*. Begin by performing this exercise for 30 seconds, and work your way up to one minute.

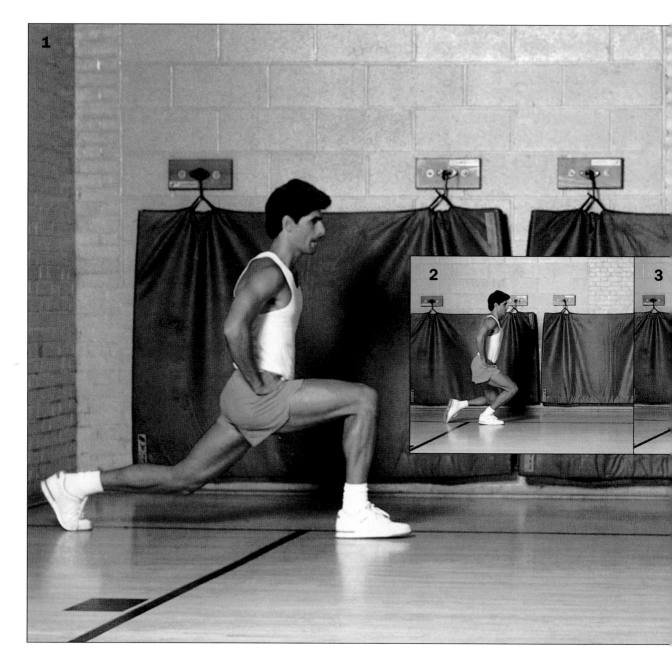

Split Squat Walk

Stand with your hands on your hips and your right leg forwards, forming
90-degree angles at the hip and knee, and your left leg extended behind you
with your left knee bent (1). Walk forwards without raising or leaning your
upper body as you progress (2, 3). Complete the stride cycle by regaining the
starting position (4, 5). Perform this walk for a distance of about 3 metres at
first; increase your distance to 9 metres.

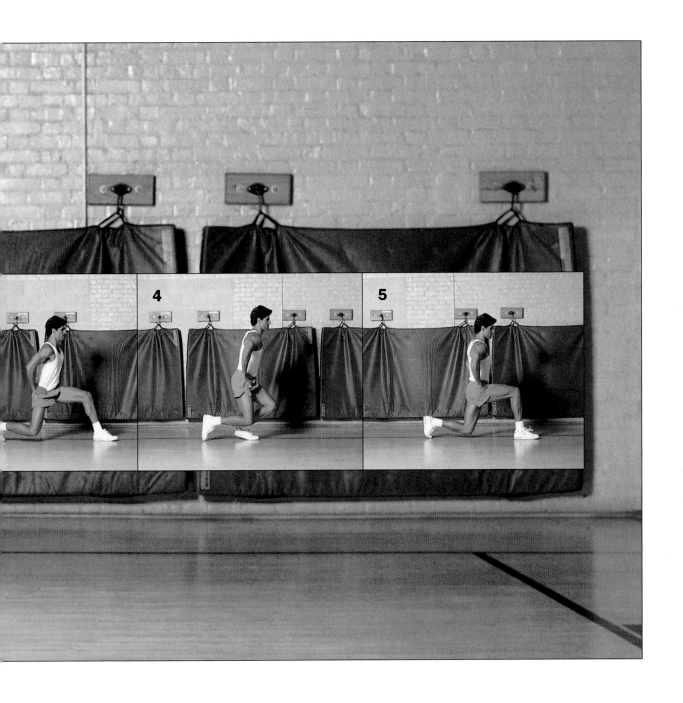

Double-Leg Tuck Jump

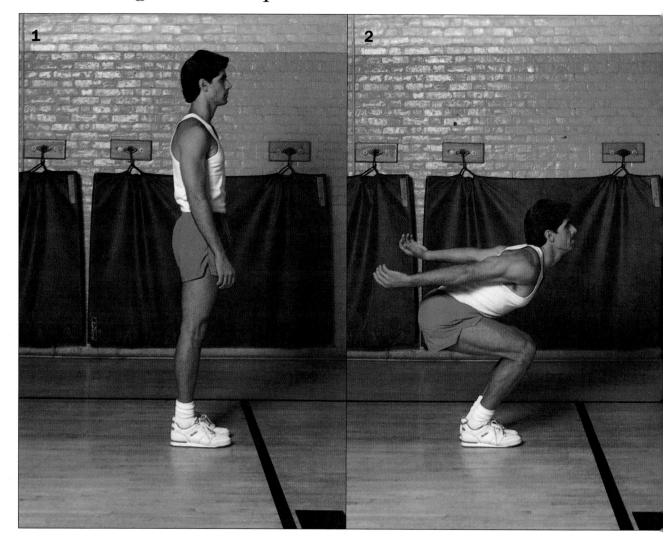

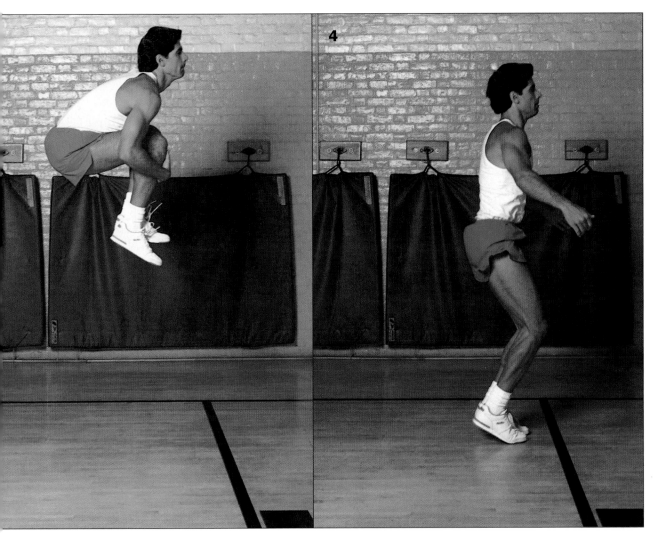

Stand with your feet shoulder-width apart and your arms at your sides (1). Bend forwards at the knees and waist with your arms extended behind you (2). Jump straight up, extending your legs, and at the same time swing your arms forwards. Then bring your knees up until your thighs are parallel to the floor and grasp your knees briefly with both hands (3). Straighten your legs to land (4).

Split Squat Jump

Stand with your hands on your hips and, keeping your back straight, lunge your right knee forwards to form a right angle and extend your left leg behind you (1). Dip on the spot so that your knee lifts about 15 centimetres from the floor, then launch yourself upwards forcefully (2). Land in the starting position (3).

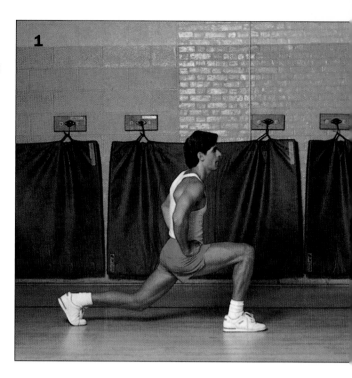

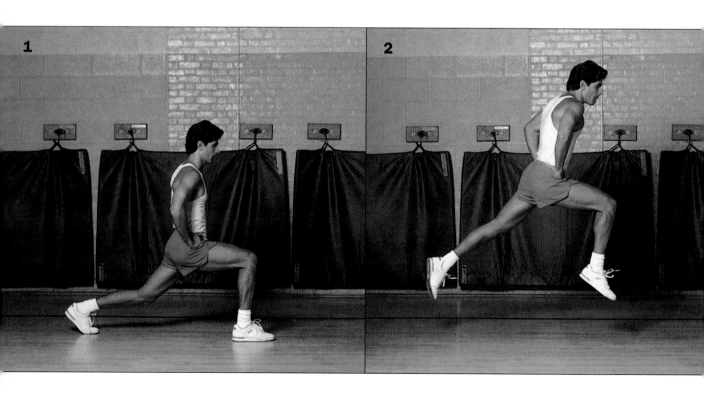

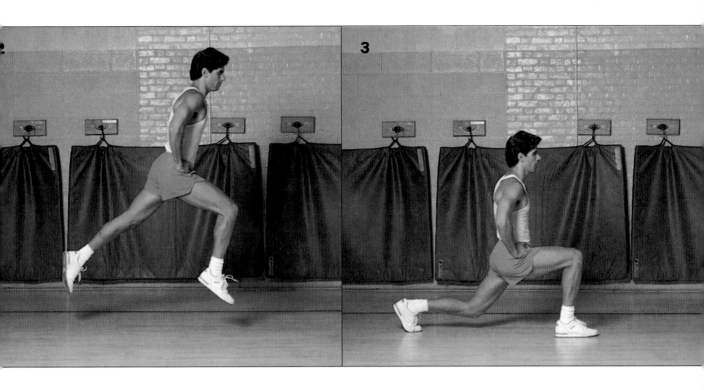

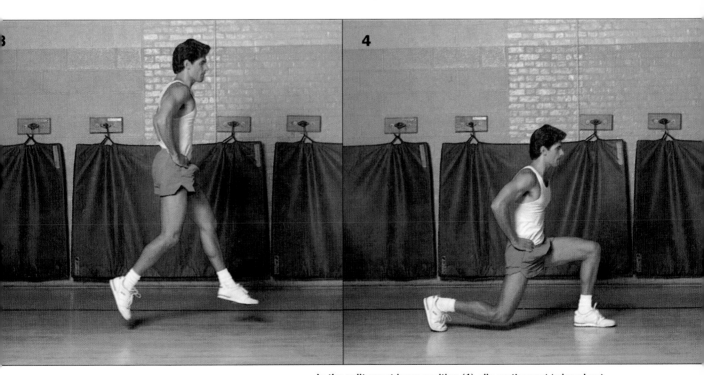

In the split squat jump position (1), dip on the spot twice about 15 centimetres from the floor and then launch yourself upwards (2), switching the positions of your legs at the peak of the jump (3). Land in the starting position with your left leg forwards (4).

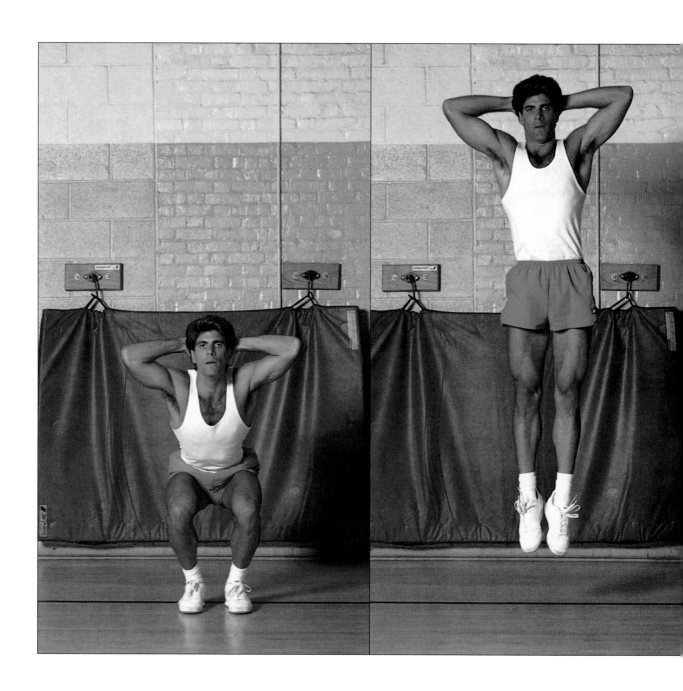

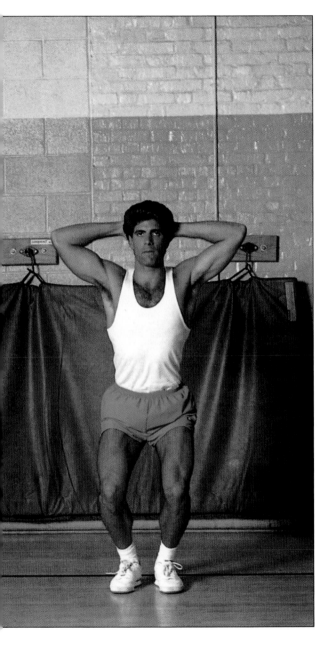

Squat Jump

Stand with your feet shoulder-width apart and your fingers interlocked behind your head. Squat so that your knees are flexed *(far left)*. Jump straight up in the air as fast as you can *(centre)*. Land in the starting position *(left)*.

Standing Broad Jump

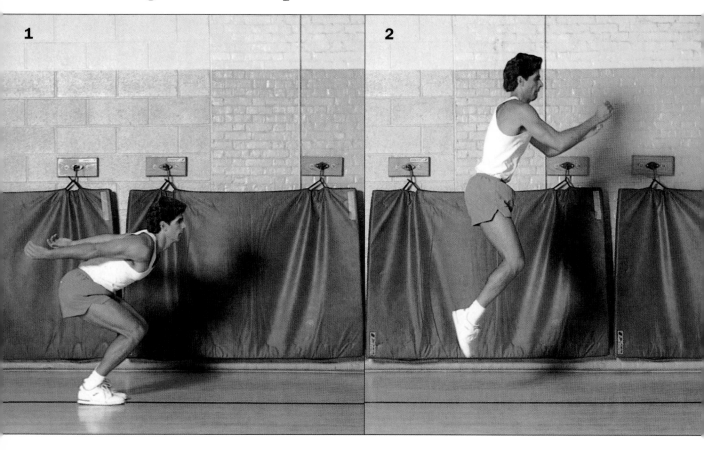

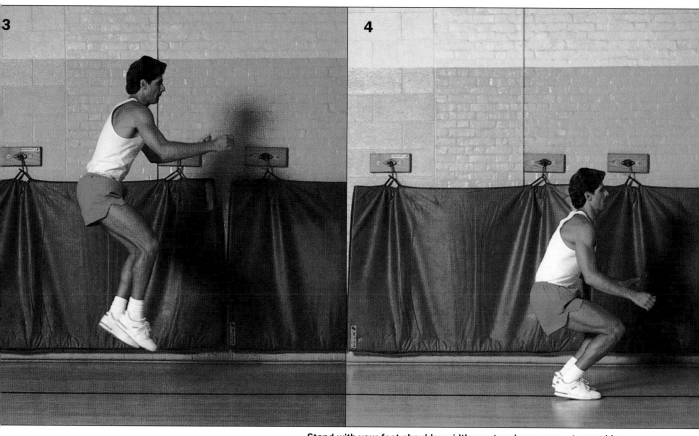

Stand with your feet shoulder-width apart and your arms at your sides. Bend forwards at the waist and knees, with your arms extended behind you (1). Jump up and forwards as far as you can by extending your legs, and swing your arms forwards (2). Lift your knees, bringing your feet forwards (3), and land with your knees and hips flexed (4).

Cone Hops

With your feet shoulder-width apart, stand with your arms at your sides and your knees bent slightly *(below)*. Jump up and forwards over the first cone by tucking your knees so that your thighs are roughly parallel to the floor *(below, right)*. Land with your hips and knees flexed slightly *(opposite)*. Immediately take off again and jump forwards over the second cone. Repeat until you have jumped over all the cones.

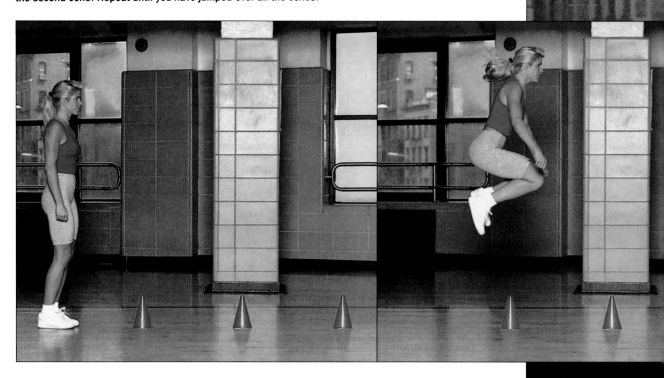

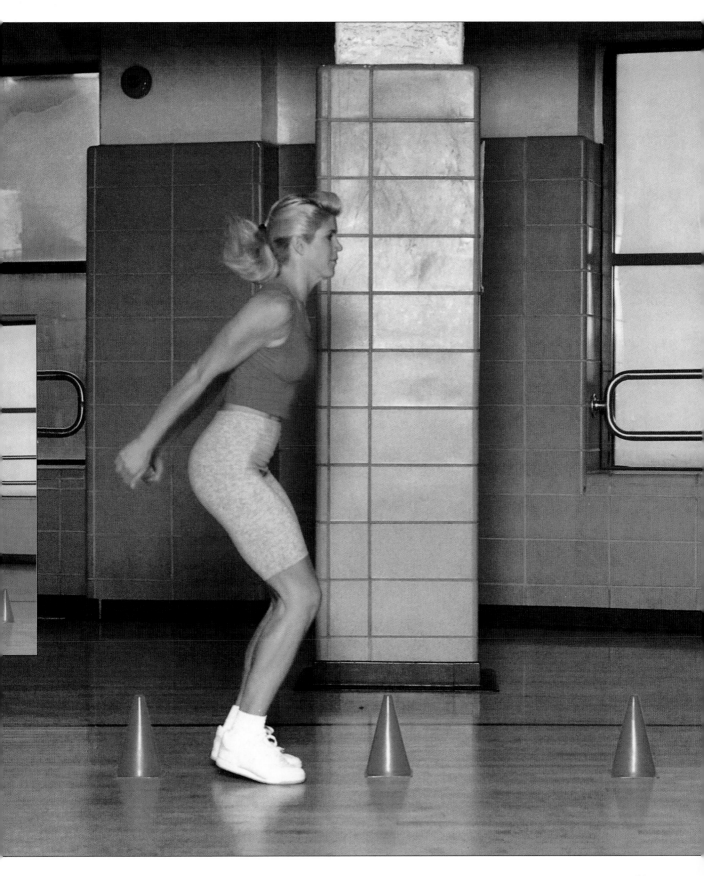

Lateral Cone Hops

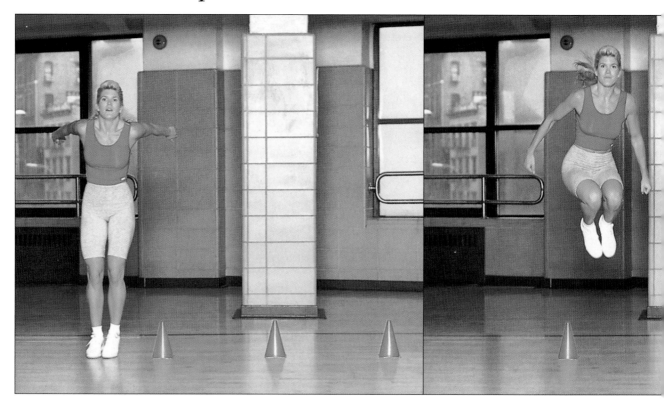

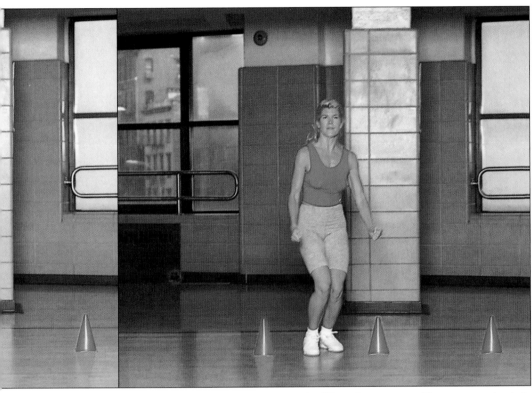

Stand to the right of a 15-centimetre cone with your arms extended behind you *(above, left)*. Jump up and sideways over the first cone, tucking your knees up so that your thighs are at least parallel to the floor *(above, centre)*. Land with your hips and knees flexed slightly *(above)*. Immediately take off again, jumping sideways over the next cone. Continue until you have jumped over all the cones.

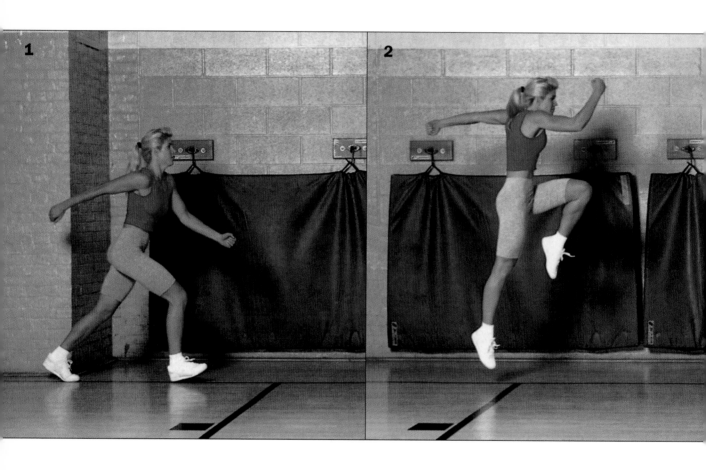

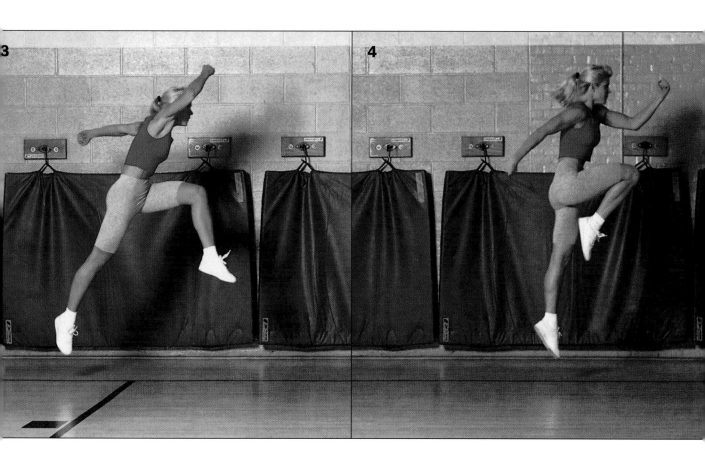

Power Skipping

From a standing position, step forwards with your right leg while swinging your left arm forwards (1). Raise your left leg, bending your knee, as you swing your right arm up forcefully, skipping forwards into the air (2, 3). Land flat-footed on your left leg and immediately skip upwards with your right leg and left arm (4). Try to attain maximum height.

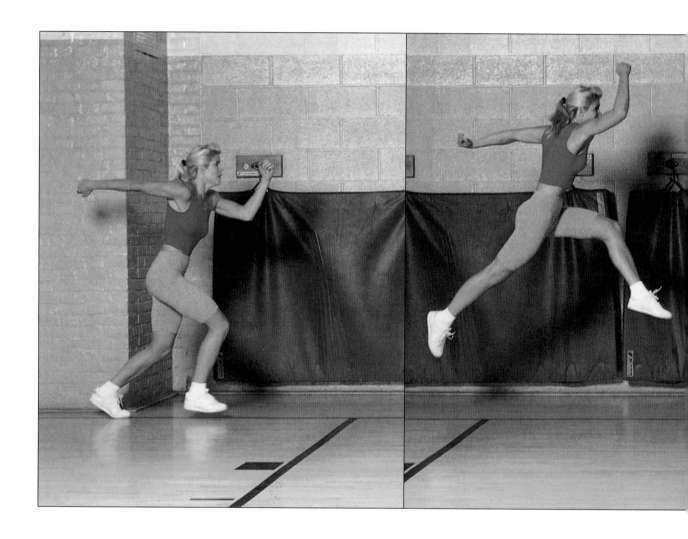

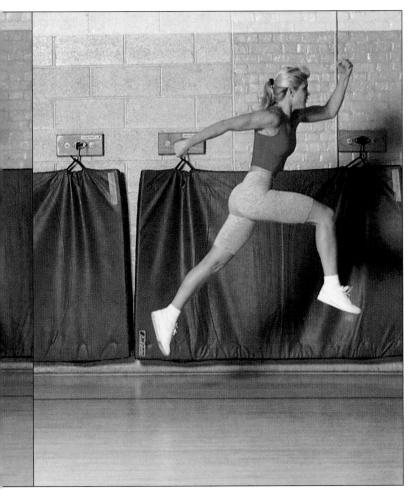

Bounding

Step forwards with your right leg as you swing your left arm forwards *(far left)*. Then leap up and forwards by driving your left leg and right arm into the air *(centre)*; pretend you are floating. Land flat-footed on your left leg and immediately drive your right leg and left arm forwards *(left)*.

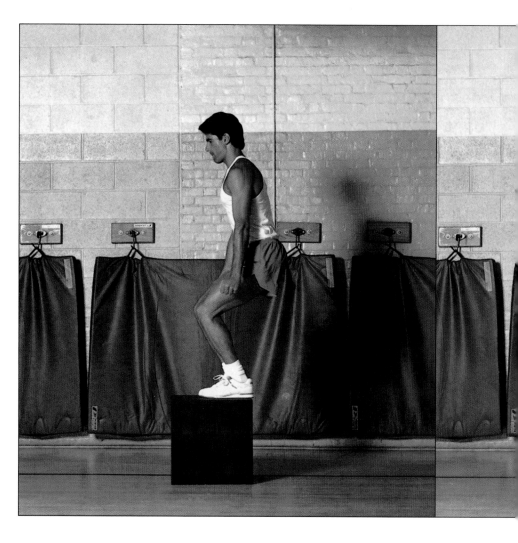

Box Routines

To build leaping power, you can step from or jump up on to a raised surface. Athletes who regularly train with plyometrics use wooden boxes that are padded and strong enough to support at least three times their weight. But you can also use a step or a sturdy bench as long as it is of sufficient height and width. An exercise mat or grass will provide cushioning for landing. For information about equipment, see the box on page 57.

To decide on the height of the box or other jumping surface, perform the jump-and-reach test. Stand beside a wall and, holding a piece of chalk, mark the highest point you can reach. Then jump as high as you can and reach up to mark the wall; the difference between the marks is your vertical jump height. You should just be able to reach your vertical jump height when performing the in-depth jump shown on page 80. Start with a 20-centimetre box. If

you can reach your jump height, try a 30-centimetre box. If you can still reach your jump height, try a box of 45 centimetres. If you cannot reach your jump height, use the 30-centimetre box; if you can reach, try a box that is 15 centimetres higher.

Be especially careful performing the in-depth jumps shown on pages 80-83. They are difficult as well as potentially injurious, and you should be in peak condition before you consider attempting them.

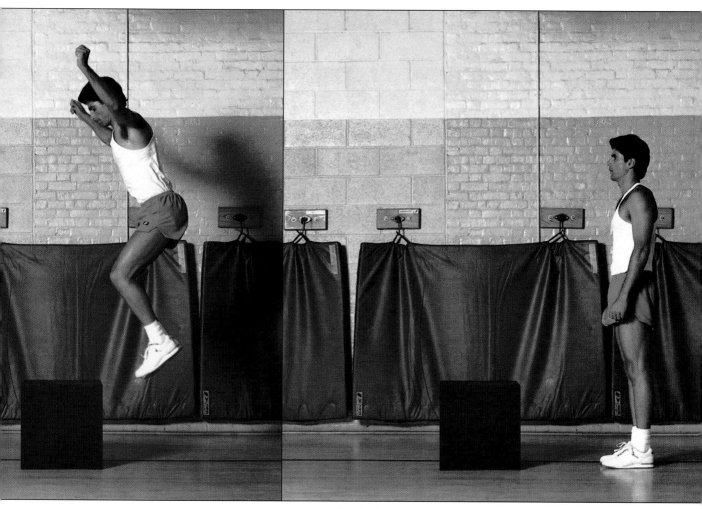

Stand relaxed, facing a box *(above)*. Bending at the hips and knees, use your arms as you jump up and on to the box *(above, centre)*. Land on your feet with your waist, hips and knees flexed *(above, left)*.

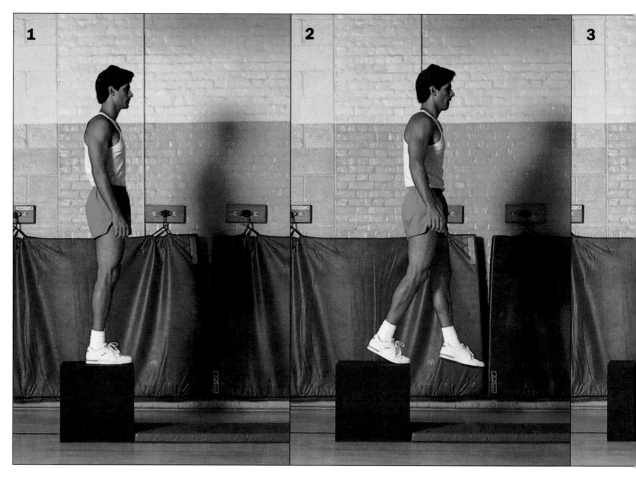

In-Depth Jump

Stand on top of the box (1), then step down on to a mat or grass (2), bending at the waist, hips and knees with your arms behind you as you land (3). Immediately jump up as high as you can, using your arms to help power yourself (4). Flex at your hips and knees as you land (5).

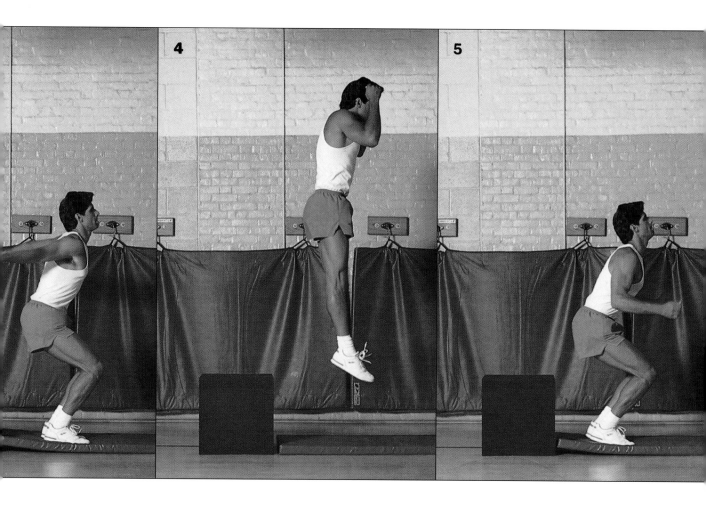

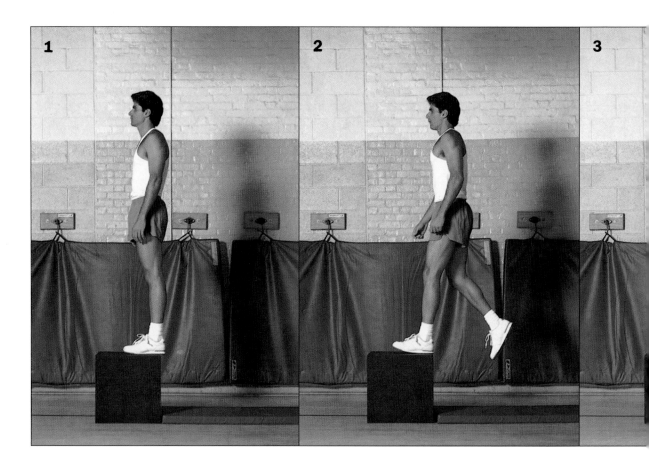

Reverse In-Depth Jump

Stand on the box (1), then step backwards with your right foot (2). Take especial care when performing this stage of the exercise, as you are acting unsighted. Flex your knees as you land and bring your arms behind you (3). Jump up forcefully as fast as you can, using your arms (4). Land with your knees and hips flexed (5).

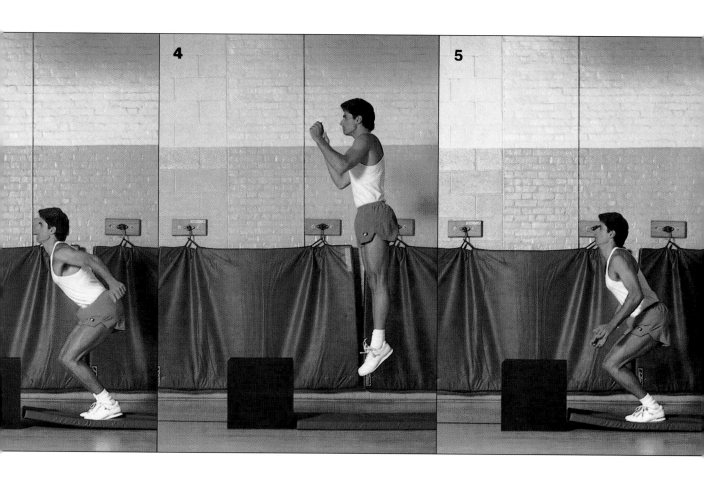

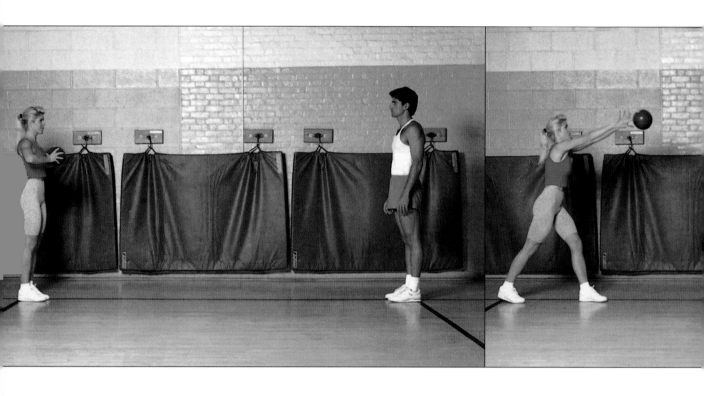

The Upper Body

Plyometric exercises for the upper body are usually performed with a medicine ball that weighs between 1.5 and 7 kilograms. Throwing the medicine ball requires a total-body effort, and it is necessary for all your muscles to be strong if your throw is to be powerful and sufficient to carry the ball forwards and upwards.

For most of these exercises, you need to throw the ball by stepping forwards first. Then you must transfer the force from your legs, through your body and into your arms. Some exercises eliminate the need to step forwards first, but the transfer of force from your torso to your arms is always necessary to complete the activity properly and effectively.

Select a medicine ball sufficiently heavy to make you work hard, but not one that is so burdensome as to hamper your form.

You will find that the exercises require you to put your upper body through a greater range of motion than would be needed to perform similar throwing movements in various sports. This exaggerated range of motion overloads your muscles, as does increasing the weight of the medicine ball. The idea is similar to that of rapidly stretching the muscles to elicit the myotatic reflex (*see page 56 for a description*).

The exercises shown on pages 86-91 are best performed with a partner, but you can do them unassisted; the exercises on pages 84-85 and 92-95 cannot be performed without a partner. Choose someone with roughly the same strength and endurance as yourself so that you both get a good workout from the exercises.

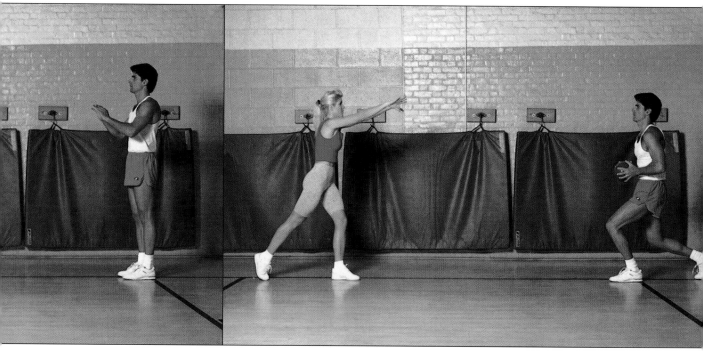

CHEST PASS Stand about 3 metres away from your partner. Hold a medicine ball at chest level *(above, left)*. Step forwards as you pass the ball to your partner, extending your arms at chest level *(above, centre)*. As soon as you let go of the ball, turn your hands downwards *(above)*.

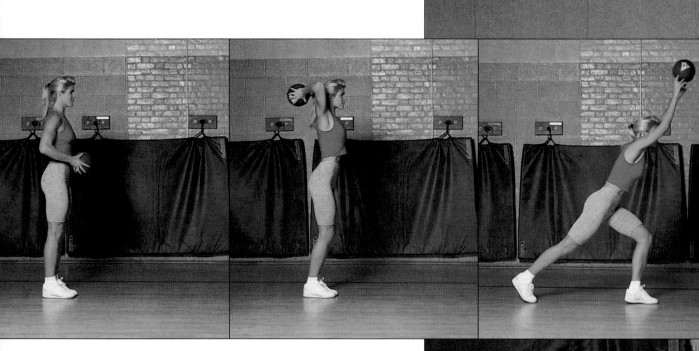

Overhead Pass

Hold a medicine ball at waist level *(above, left)*. Raise the ball back behind your head and flex your knees as you prepare to throw *(above, centre)*. Step forwards with your left leg and throw the ball by bringing it overhead *(above, right)*. Finish the throw by extending your arms and turning your palms downwards *(opposite)*. Alternate legs when you repeat the exercise.

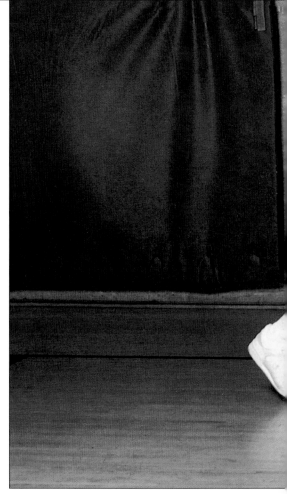

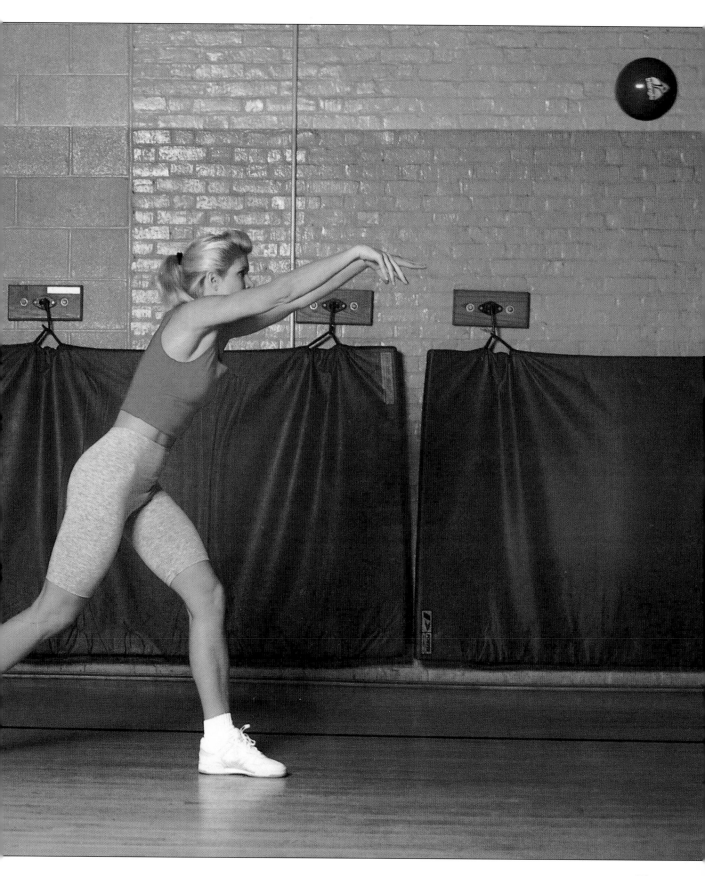

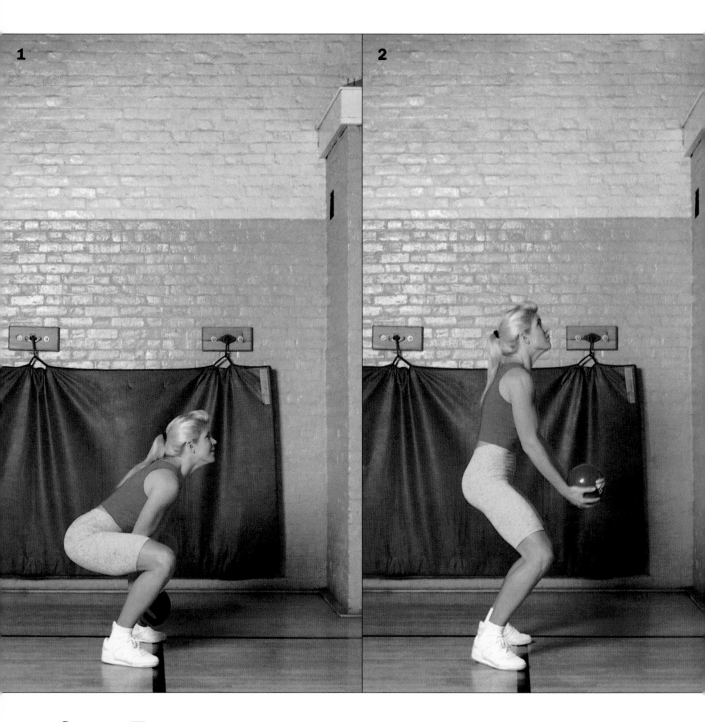

Scoop Toss

Stand up straight while holding a medicine ball cupped in your hands. Flex your hips and knees until your thighs are parallel to the floor, bringing the ball between your legs (1). Raise the ball as you rise up and forwards (2), extending your body as you toss the ball upwards (3). Land with your arms at your sides and your knees flexed (4).

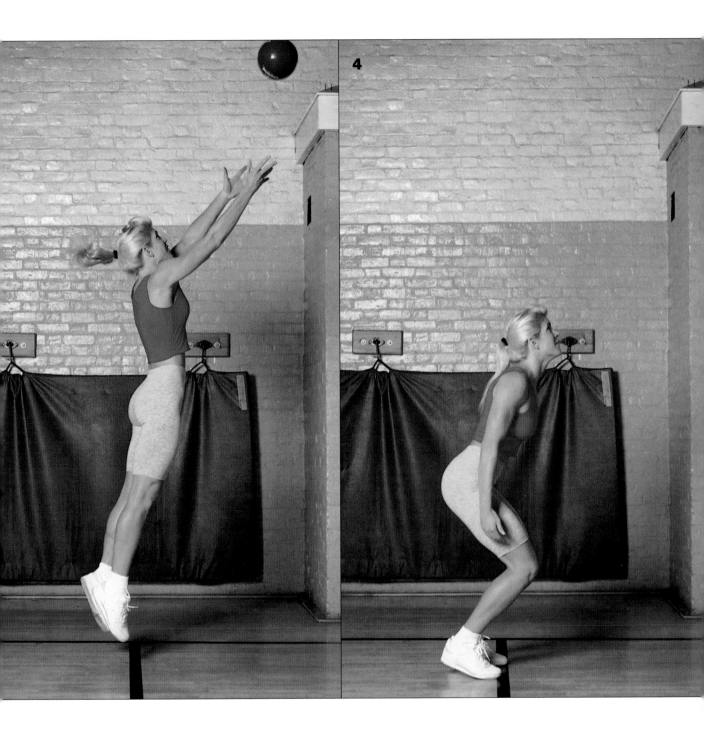

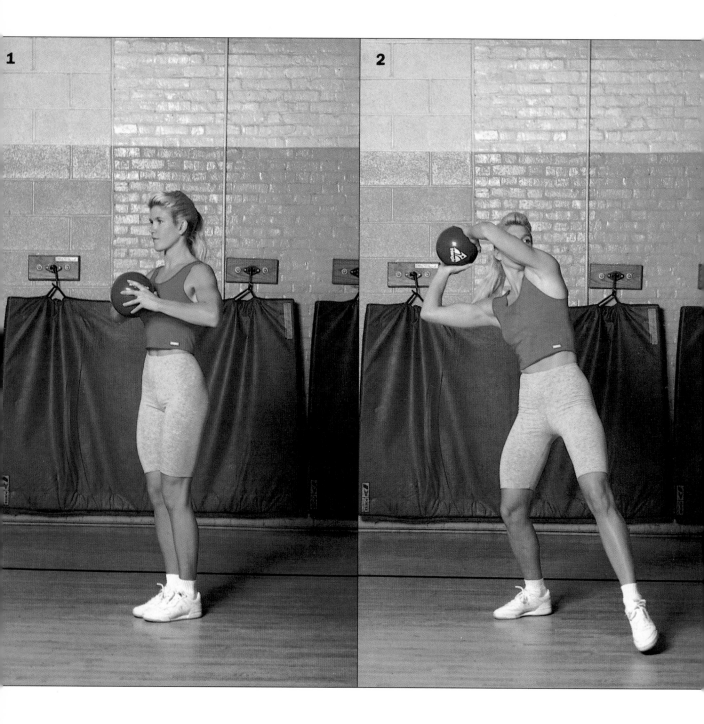

Diagonal Pass

Stand with your knees flexed and your feet slightly apart, holding a
medicine ball at chest level (1). Bring the ball back over your right
shoulder as you lean backwards (2). Step forwards with your left leg as
you throw the ball diagonally over your right shoulder. The ball should
be in line with your right shoulder and your left hip (3). Your torso
should be bent forwards and turned slightly to the left with your palms
outwards (4). Alternate passes from both sides as you do the exercise.

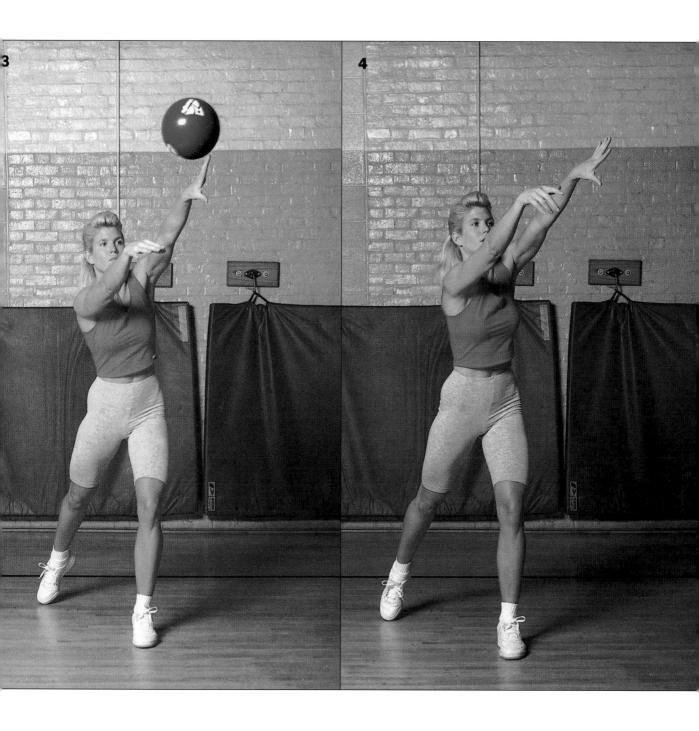

Medicine Ball Sit-Ups

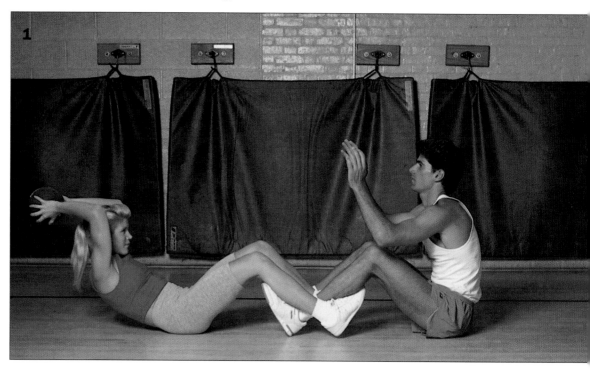

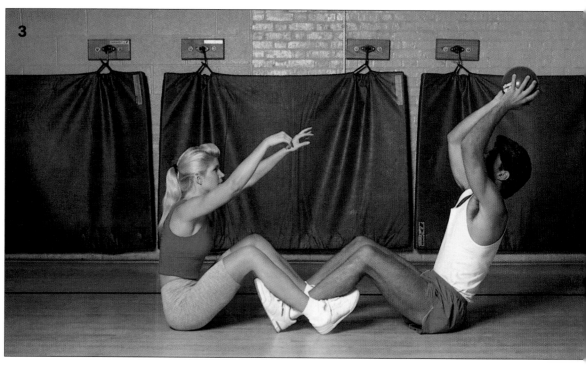

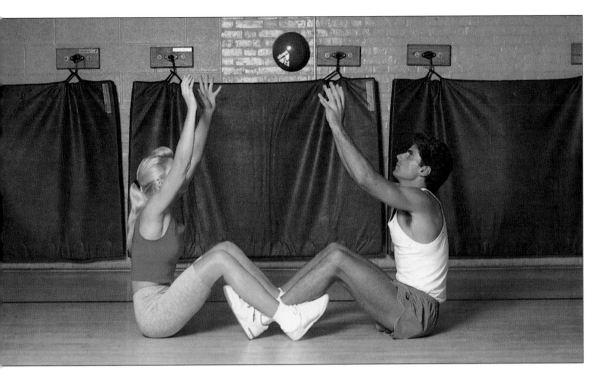

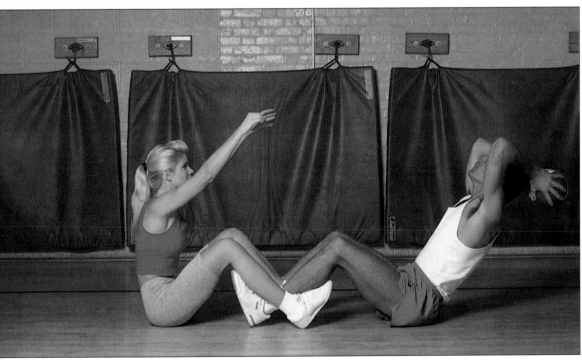

Sit facing your partner with your knees and hips flexed and your legs interlocked. Hold a medicine ball overhead, leaning backwards until your back is nearly on the floor (1). Perform a sit-up, keeping your arms locked in the starting position, and release the ball when your torso is vertical (2). The force of the throw comes from your abdominals, not your arms. Your partner should catch the ball overhead, contracting his abdominals to prevent himself from falling backwards (3). Then your partner performs a sit-up before throwing the ball (4). Avoid this exercise if you suffer from lower back pain.

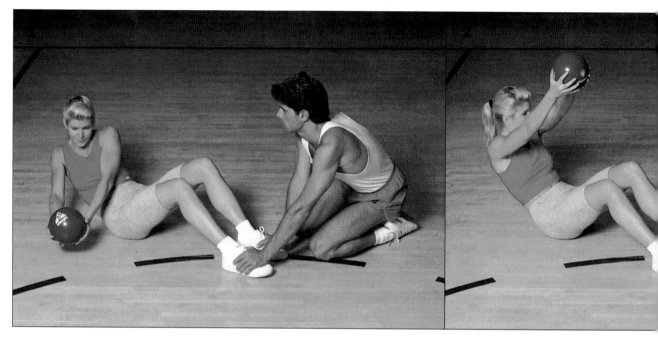

Diagonal Twist

Hold a medicine ball cupped in your hands while sitting on the floor with your hips and knees flexed. Your partner secures your feet as you lean backwards, forming a 90-degree angle at your waist. Twist your torso with your arms extended to the right a few centimetres above the floor (1). Raise the ball above your chest as you twist to your left (2). Continue to twist as you lower the ball to your left (3). Then twist to the right again, raising the ball (4), until you reach the starting position (5). Avoid this exercise if you suffer from lower back pain.

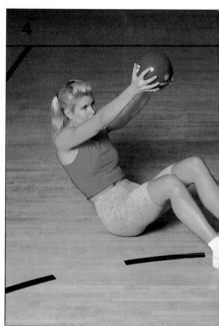

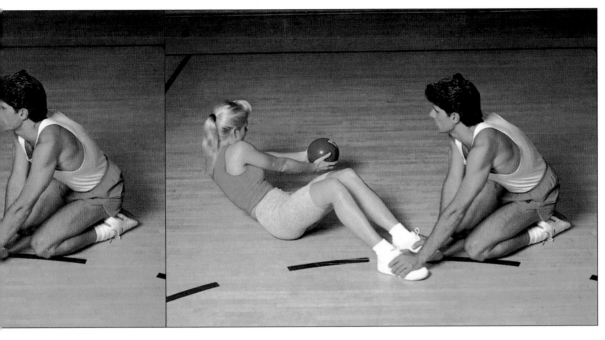

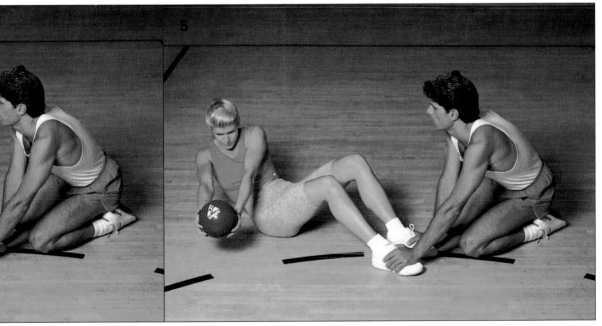

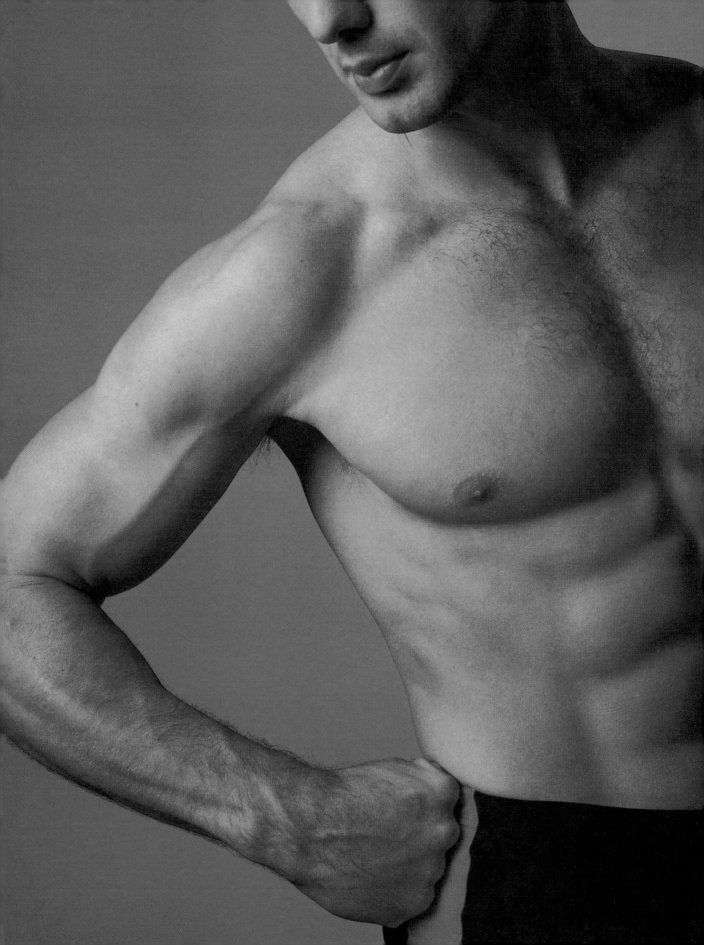

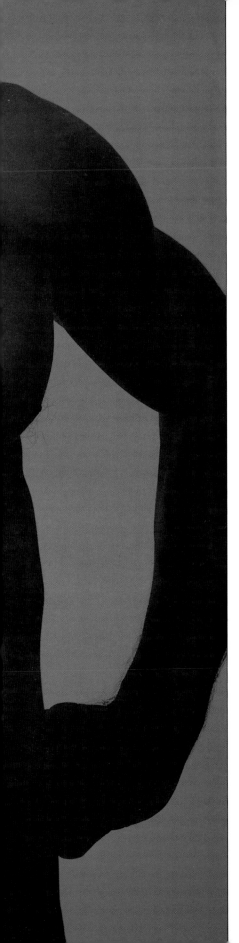

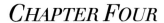
Circuit Training

A military-style workout for strengthening your muscles and cardiovascular system

There is no master exercise that maintains all the various aspects of fitness. Running, for instance, is a great aerobic conditioner but does little to improve muscle strength. Chin-ups increase both muscle power and endurance in your arms and shoulders, but contribute nothing to benefit either your flexibility or your aerobic capacity. Recognizing this problem, researchers based at the University of Leeds developed circuit training — a method of conditioning that develops muscular strength and endurance, flexibility and aerobic fitness in a single programme of exercises that are performed in a particular sequence.

The original circuits consisted of a series of six to 10 stations set up in a gymnasium or on a field. The circuit trainer would run between the stations, which were spaced apart at varying distances, and perform the exercises — for example, 25 sit-ups or 50 jumping jacks — at each stop. The longer the distance between stations, the greater the aerobic benefit the exerciser derived from performing the circuit.

Similarly, you could enhance the strength-building component by increasing the number of stations that involve muscle development.

Although slow to catch on at first, the idea of circuit training was marketed by several companies that developed circuit-training courses. These courses, laid out along running trails, resemble military obstacle courses, with nine to 18 stations that contain simple apparatus for performing warm-ups, and such exercises as jumping jacks, chin-ups, sit-ups, push-ups and balancing routines. Many circuits include not only aerobic and strength-building exercises, but also routines for co-ordination and stretching that provide a workout that encompasses all the elements of fitness. One manufacturer in America has installed more than 3,500 circuit courses in public parks, schools, hotels, office parks and military bases. In one survey of corporate employees who used a circuit-training course, many reported that they lost weight, felt better, slept more soundly and had more energy as a result.

Since you must do something different at every station, the tedium of an extended bout of repeated exercise is relieved by circuit training. In a well-designed circuit, you start slowly to ensure an adequate warm-up, and you perform exercises of gradually increasing difficulty. The stations are arranged to provide a specific sequence of exercise for the upper body, the abdominals and the legs. Finally, the intensity of the workout is gradually reduced to cool you down safely.

You do not need a formal or permanent course of stations to derive the benefits of circuit training. The regimen represented in this chapter involves a minimum amount of equipment, yet it provides a physically challenging series of stations for a full-body workout tailored to your own needs and pace. The exercises are based on training routines used in the United States Military Academy at West Point, New York State, and many of them are arranged in mini-circuits, in which each station consists of a multiple set of exercises designed to enhance a specific component of fitness — muscular endurance, for instance — and condition a particular part of your body.

It is not necessary or even desirable to perform all of these circuits every day; rather, a workout should consist of three or four of them. You can also incorporate one or more of the mini-circuits at the conclusion of an aerobic workout, such as a long run or a stationary bicycle session. In each circuit, you should perform every exercise that is included. Then, for your next workout, choose a different combination of circuits. When you select a set of circuits, choose a combination of moderate and difficult exercises that condition both your upper and lower body. This allows you to derive the greatest benefit from the routine without becoming exhausted. Also, alternate upper and lower body exercises within each workout. (For a guide to circuit combinations, see the box on the opposite page.)

You can perform many of these circuits indoors by jogging on the spot or alternating jumping jacks between stations, or you can circuit train in your back garden or around your neighbourhood. If you live

Circuit Combinations

It is not necessary to incorporate every circuit shown in this chapter in every training session. For variety — as well as to give yourself a rest — you can omit some circuits or substitute them for others on alternate days. No matter what combination you use, however, you should always include a five to 10-minute warm-up and stretching session at the beginning of each workout, and a five-minute cool-down at the end. In addition, you should also perform the abdominal curls and lifts (pages 104-109), or a few of the exercises, at least three or four times per week. The following is a sample weekly schedule that employs a hard day/easy day concept, which means you alternate days of strenuous exercise with ones that are relatively easy.

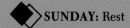 **MONDAY:** Warm-ups and Stretches *(pages 100-103)*, 20-minute run, Two-for-One Callisthenics *(pages 122-127)*, Horizontal Ladder Circuit *(pages 118-121)*, Lifts and Curls *(pages 104-109)*, cool-down.

TUESDAY: Warm-ups and Stretches *(pages 100-103)*, Leg Workers Circuit *(pages 114-117)*, Push-Up Circuit *(pages 132-137)*, Lifts and Curls *(pages 104-109)*, cool-down.

WEDNESDAY: Warm-ups and Stretches *(pages 100-103)*, Hill Running *(pages 112-113)*, Sandbag Circuit *(pages 128-131)*, cool-down.

THURSDAY: Warm-ups and Stretches *(pages 100-103)*, Rope Climbing *(pages 138-141)*, 20 to 30-minute run or Leg Workers Circuit *(pages 114-117)*, Two-for-One Callisthenics *(pages 122-127)*, twistie and straight curls *(pages 106-107)*, cool-down.

FRIDAY: Warm-ups and Stretches *(pages 100-103)*, Stair Circuit *(pages 110-111)*, Push-up Circuit *(pages 132-137)*, Lifts and Curls *(pages 104-109)*, cool-down.

SATURDAY: Warm-ups and Stretches *(pages 100-103)*, 30-minute jog, Horizontal Ladder Circuit *(pages 118-121)*, Lifts and Curls *(pages 104-109)*, cool-down.

SUNDAY: Rest

near a school with a playground, for instance, you might be able to make use of the horizontal ladder as a station to perform pull-ups and other exercises *(see pages 118-121)*. If a nearby park has terraced steps, you can use these as a station for building leg endurance; or you could use a local sports stadium *(see pages 110-111)*.

Many of the exercises that follow are quite strenuous. In order to work out at a level intense enough to achieve fitness benefits, yet not so strenuous that you become injured, you must listen to your body and monitor how you feel. If you find that performing a particular mini-circuit leaves you feeling exhausted and sore, you can cut back to a more manageable level. In addition, if there are any exercises in this chapter that are difficult for you to perform safely, such as the supine leg lifts on page 106 or the rope climb on pages 138-141, leave them out entirely or perform them at a lower intensity until you have attained sufficient strength and agility.

Warm-Ups and Stretches

The warm-up exercises and stretches shown on these two pages and the following two are specific movements designed to prepare your body for the more vigorous activities that follow. Some of the later routines are extremely strenuous and require a maximum range of motion in your joints and muscles. In order to avoid injury and derive the greatest benefit from circuit training, it is essential that you warm up thoroughly.

Once your body begins warming up, oxygen exchange between the blood and the muscles is enhanced, metabolic chemical reactions take place at a faster rate and nervous impulses fire more quickly. Moreover, warming up decreases the internal friction of your muscles and joints.

Stretching after you have warmed up increases muscle flexibility and helps minimize the risk of musculo-skeletal injury. Most experts agree that tight and inflexible muscles are more prone to pulls, tears and other stresses and injuries.

Begin your warm-up session with one minute of marching on the spot, then follow with the exercises shown on the right. When you have finished them, run on the spot for another 60 seconds before progressing to the following pages. Once you have completed the stretches shown on pages 102-103, repeat all of them again for the opposite limbs.

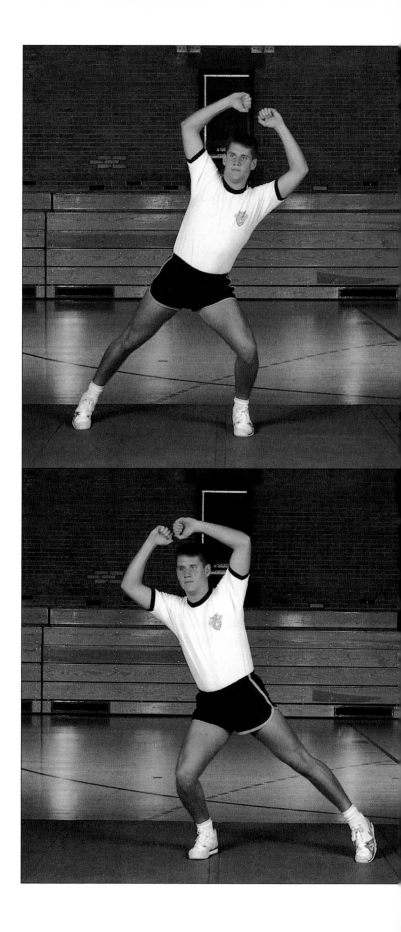

LOW-IMPACT JACKS Stand with your hands at your sides, your knees flexed slightly and your back straight. Raise your hands over your head and swing your right leg to the side *(right, above)*. Return to the starting position. Raise your hands again and swing your left leg to the side *(right)*. Repeat the exercise for 60 seconds.

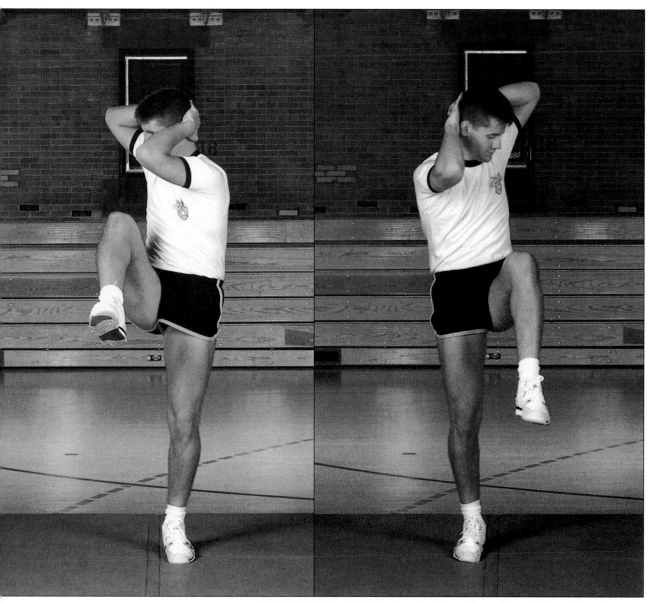

ALTERNATE KNEE LIFTS Stand erect with your knees bent slightly and interlace your fingers behind your head. Twist your torso to the right and lift your right knee towards your left elbow *(above, left)*. Return to the starting position, then twist your torso to the left and lift your left knee towards your right elbow *(above)*. Return to the starting position. Continue for 60 seconds.

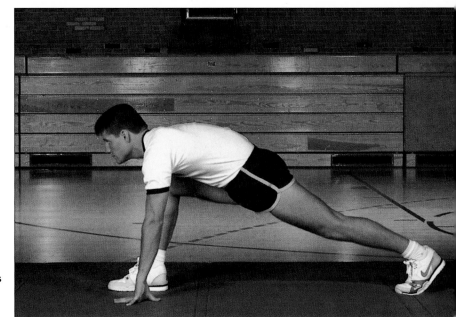

SPIDER Bend over and position your hands on the floor with your elbows inside your knees, which you should not bend more than 90 degrees. Extend your left leg to the side *(right)*. Hold for at least 10 to 15 seconds.

LUNGE From the spider position, keep your feet in place and swing your body to the right, moving your hands to both sides of your right foot *(right)*. Try to drop your hips to the floor, keeping your back leg straight. Hold for 10 to 15 seconds.

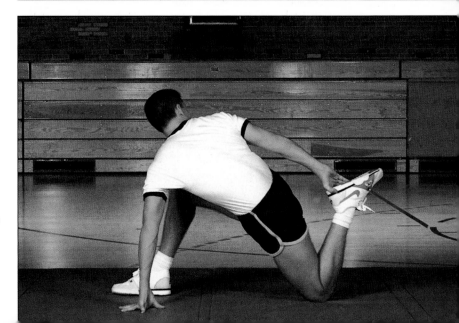

QUAD STRETCH From the lunge position, drop your left knee to the floor and grasp your left heel with your right hand. Draw your heel towards your buttocks *(right)*. Hold for 10 to 15 seconds.

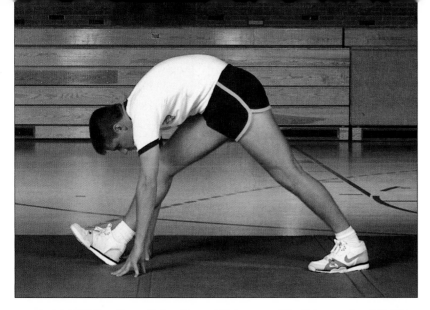

HAMSTRING STRETCH Return your right hand next to your right foot, extend your left leg and place your foot flat on the floor. Raise your right toes *(left)*. Hold the stretch for 10 to 15 seconds.

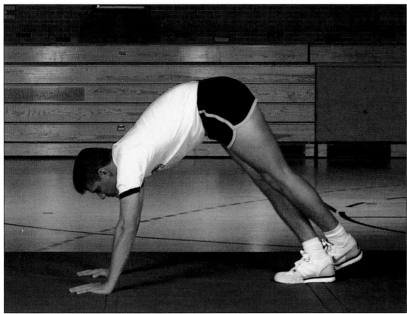

CALF STRETCH Draw your right leg back next to your left leg; place your palms flat on the floor. Swing your left foot behind your right heel and press it against the floor *(left)*. Hold for 10 to 15 seconds.

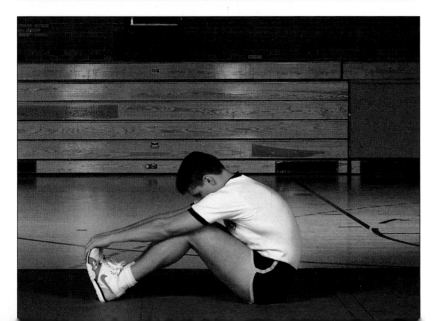

LOW BACK STRETCH Sit on the floor, draw your knees to your chest and grasp your toes *(left)*. Hold for 10 to 15 seconds. Repeat all the stretches from the beginning using the opposite limbs.

Lifts and Curls

Many people neglect their abdominal muscles when they work out. However, strong abdominals are important for good posture, and they eliminate strain on the lower back. Along with well-toned abdominals, strong hip flexor muscles, which you use to lift your knees, help to reduce the risk of lower back injuries.

The exercises on pages 104-109 will develop muscular strength and conditioning in the abdominals and hip flexors. They should be performed three or four times a week, as outlined in the box on page 99. If any exercise causes back pain, stop immediately and reduce the number of repetitions in future workouts until you build up more abdominal strength. Perform the exercises in the order presented so that the upper-abdominal stabilizing fibres do not become fatigued.

LEG LIFTS Hang from a bar with your hands shoulder-width apart. Lift your knees towards your chest, keeping your lower back rounded so that your pelvis is rotated forwards *(inset)*. Begin with 15 bent-knee lifts. Rest for 10 seconds and repeat. As you become stronger, straighten your legs to increase the effort *(right)*. When you can, perform 10 straight-leg lifts, then five with bent knees. Rest for 10 to 15 seconds and repeat.

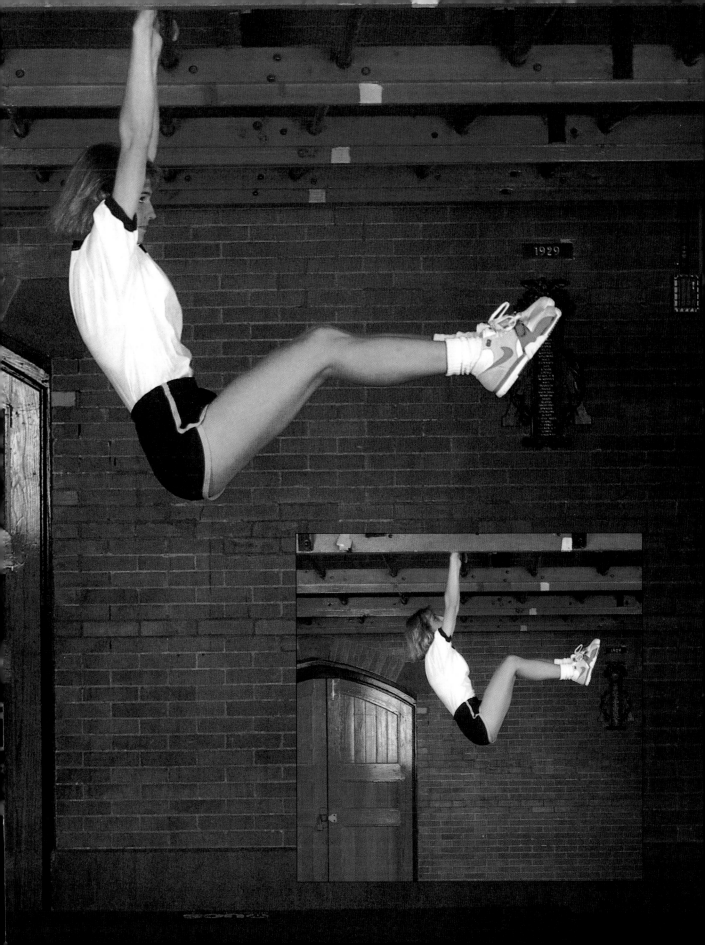

LIFTS AND CURLS
(continued)

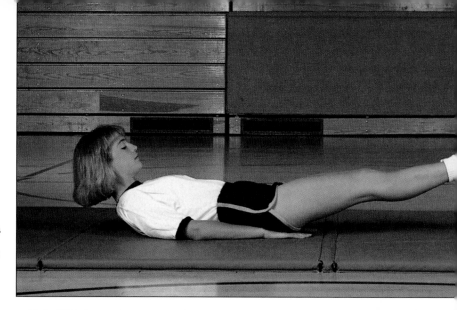

SUPINE LEG LIFTS Lie on an exercise mat with your hands under your pelvis to prevent arching. Lift your head and raise your legs 30 centimetres off the floor *(right)*. Rock your pelvis and raise your legs 45 centimetres off the floor *(far right)*. Alternate between 30 and 45 centimetres for 25 reps. Rest for 10 seconds; repeat 20 times. Avoid this exercise if you suffer from lower back pain.

TWISTIE CURLS Lie on your back with your hands behind your head, knees bent and feet flat on the floor. Lift your head and turn your torso to the right *(right)*. Leading with your left elbow, rise into a curl and hold for a full second *(far right)*. Maintain the twist throughout the range of motion. Perform 20 reps for the left side, then repeat for the right side without resting.

STRAIGHT CURLS Remain on your back with your hands behind your head and your feet flat on the floor *(right)*. Slowly raise your shoulders off the ground no more than 15 to 20 centimetres *(far right)*. Hold for one second and return to the starting position. Perform 30 reps.

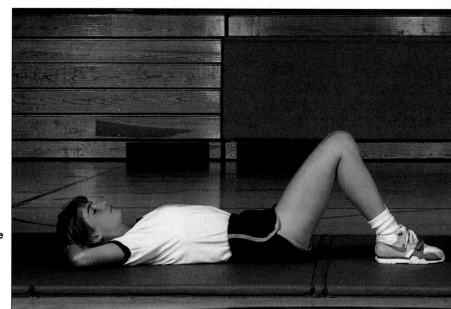

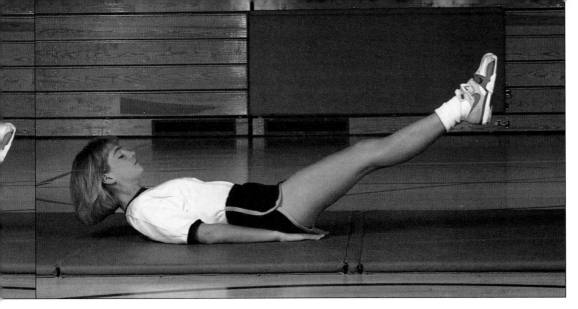

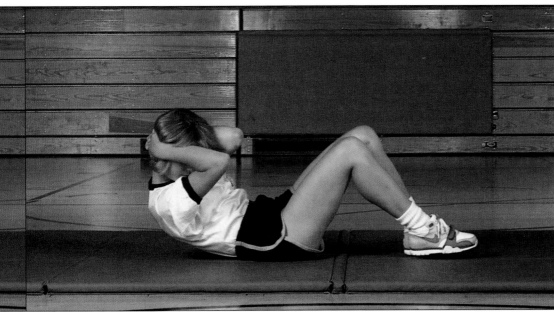

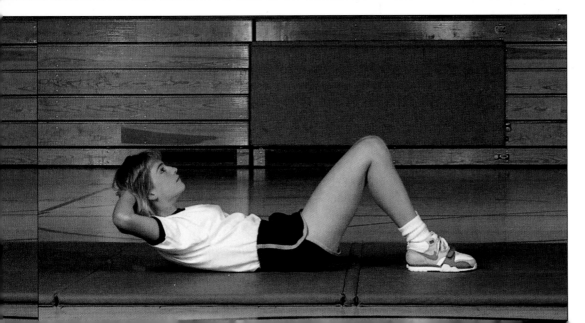

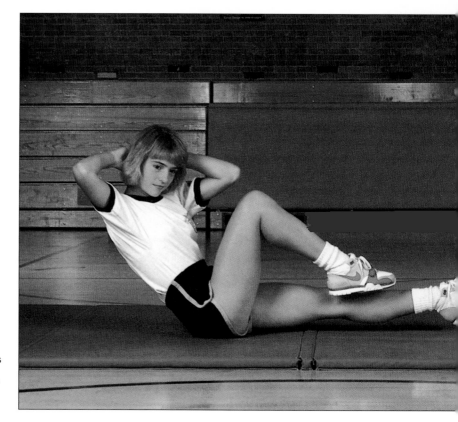

BICYCLE Keep your hands behind your head, extend your legs and sit up. Draw your right knee up and twist your body to the right, bringing your left elbow towards your knee *(right)*. Then extend your right leg, draw your left knee up and twist your right elbow towards the knee *(far right)*. Perform 30 repetitions.

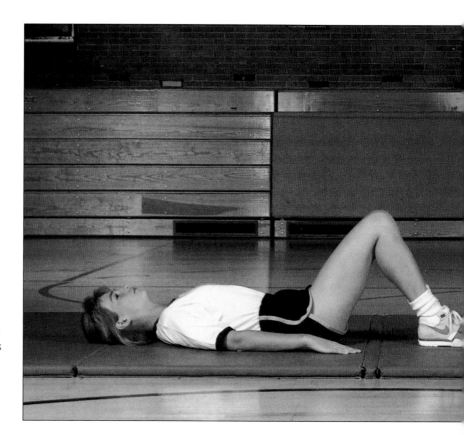

ROCKER Lie on your back with your feet flat on the floor. Place your arms at your sides with your palms down *(right)*. Rock on to your upper back and draw your knees to your chest *(far right)*; avoid placing too much weight on the neck. Hold for a second, then return to the starting position. Repeat 15 to 20 times at a moderate pace.

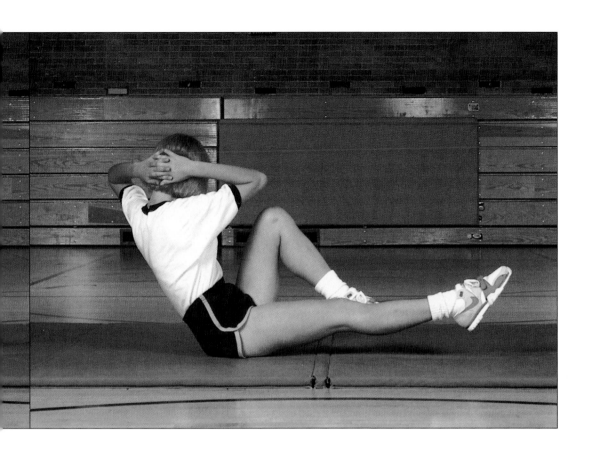

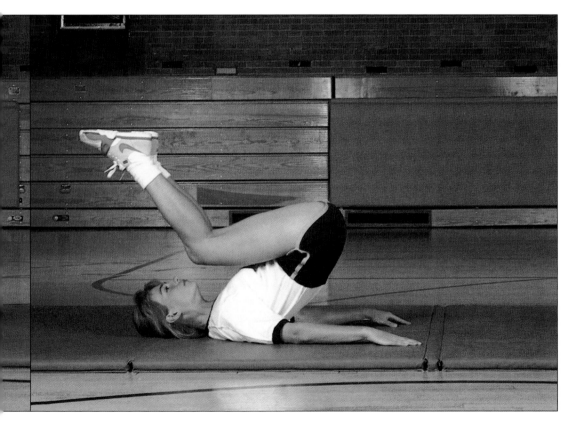

Star Circuit

According to one exercise physiologist, running up stairs is seldom incorporated in a training routine. Because most steps are the same height and most staircases rise at the same angle, they all provide about the same level of challenge. Running up stairs is a powerful exercise for the legs and helps develop both muscular endurance and cardiovascular fitness.

Find a staircase that has a landing after 18 to 24 steps, like those found in many stadiums. Do not try to run up a larger number of steps at one time, since this will provide you with too much recovery time as you jog down the stairs. Make sure you are warmed up sufficiently before you begin, then proceed with the stair-running exercises on the right. The complete circuit consists of 10 repetitions of stair running, then two reps of stair running, then two reps of stair hopping on each leg, 10 more runs, and finally, jumping up the stairs for two reps; this should take 20 minutes to complete. If you feel unsteady or dizzy at any point during the one-leg hops, stop immediately and do not continue.

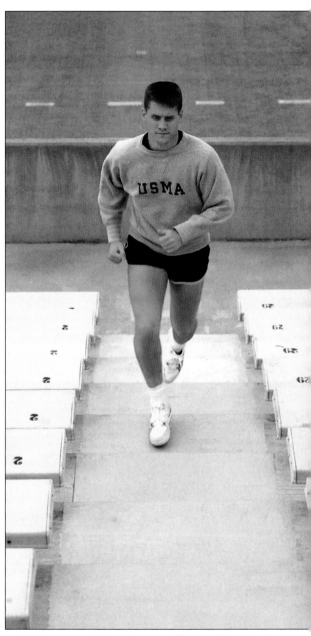

RUN Run up and down the steps 10 times. Do not push yourself too hard; but at the same time, do not rest between each repetition; pace yourself carefully so that you do not become exhausted.

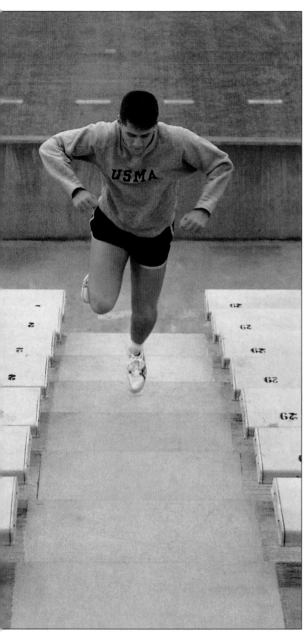

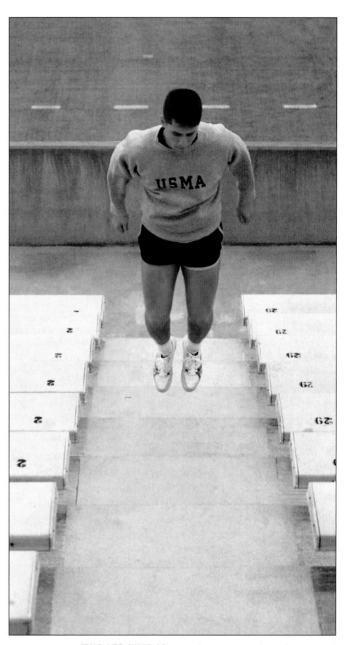

ONE-LEG HOP Hop up the stairs on your left leg and jog down on both legs; repeat. Hop up on your right leg and jog down on both legs; repeat. Then run up and down 10 times on both legs.

TWO-LEG JUMP After you have repeated running up and down the stairs 10 times on both legs, jump up the stairs with both feet together. Jog down and repeat jumping up on two feet.

Hill Running

Hills will give you about the same training benefits as running up and down stairs, except that every hill is different, providing a specific level of challenge. To ensure a good workout, find a hill that has a 10 to 12-per cent (1 in 10 to 1 in 8) incline and measure off a distance up the hill of approximately 300 metres.

To perform your hill workout, sprint up the 300 metres and then walk or jog back down. Repeat this six to eight times, and then add reps until you can perform it 10 to 12 times. In a beginner's programme, you may run up the hill in one minute and 30 to 45 seconds, and jog or walk down it in about two minutes. As you gain strength and speed, it may take you only 1:15 to 1:30 to run up a hill.

When you run up a hill, lean forwards slightly to give yourself momentum and the sensation that you are "falling" up the hill. Pump your arms powerfully and imagine that you are using them to pull yourself up on a rope. Look at a point on the road about 10 metres in front of you rather than looking at your feet or the crest of the hill.

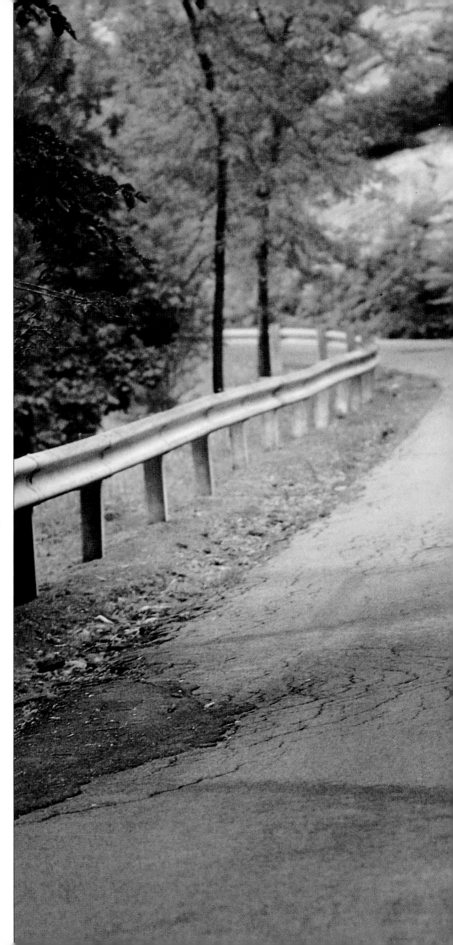

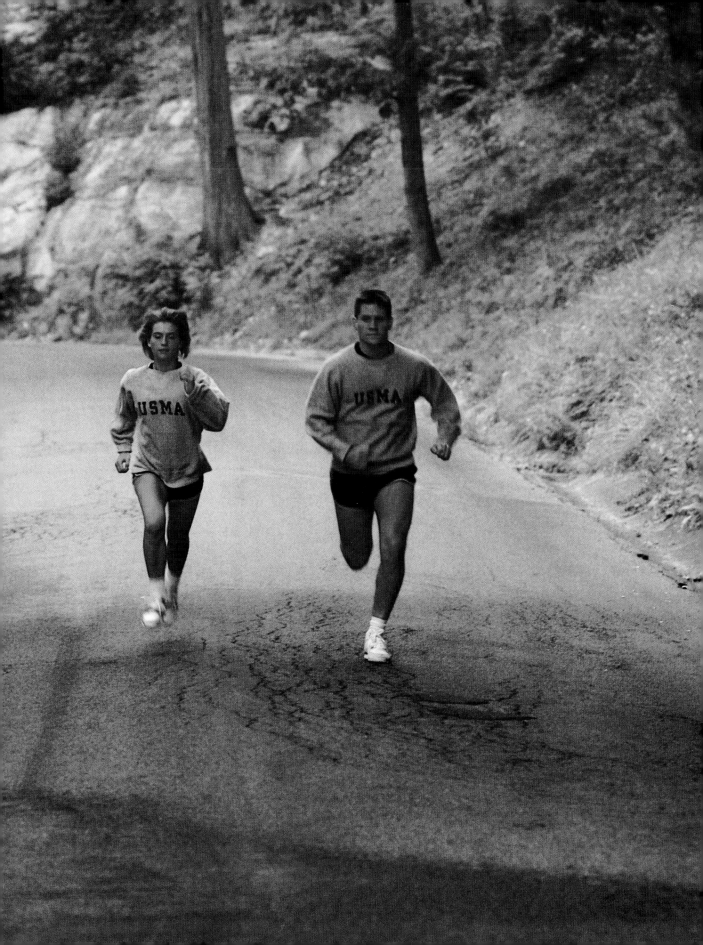

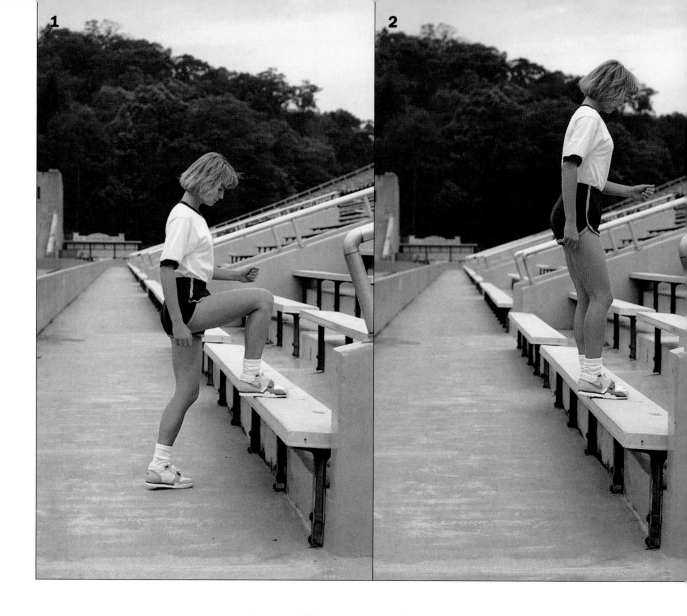

Leg Workers Circuit

This circuit of exercises will help develop muscular endurance in the most powerful muscles of your body — the quadriceps and hamstrings, the gluteals in your buttocks and the gastrocnemius muscles in your calves. The complete circuit consists of the bench steps, sissy squats and heel raises performed continuously as shown without rest; you can do one or more sets of this circuit.

For the bench step and heel raise exercises, men should find a bench that is 40 to 45 centimetres high; most women will probably prefer a 35 to 40-centimetre bench. Make sure the bench is sturdy and will not tip when you use it. Benches in stadiums or gymnasiums are often ideal for this purpose.

Be sure that you maintain good posture throughout the circuit and do not strain your back by leaning over or arching. Again, these exercises can be strenuous. Stop immediately if you become exhausted or are in danger of losing your balance.

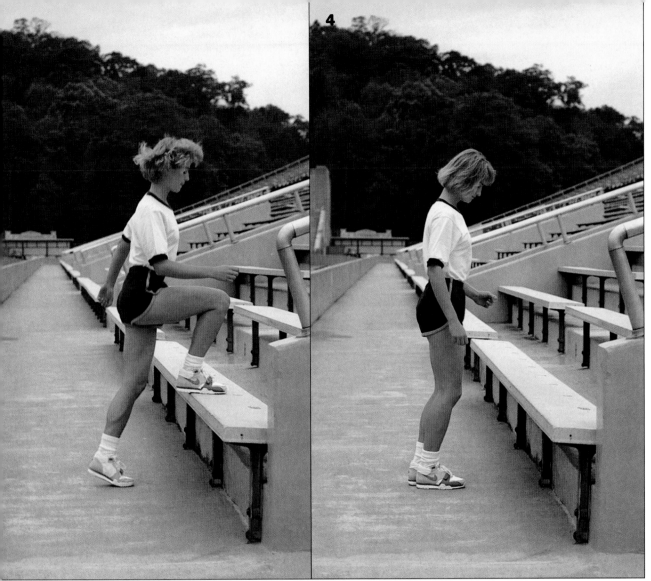

BENCH STEPS Stand in front of the bench and step up with your right foot (1). Then step up with your left (2). Step down with your left (3), and then with your right (4). In this exercise, one step is complete after both feet are on the ground in the starting position. Perform at a pace of 40 to 45 steps per minute for up to five minutes, depending on your level of fitness. Change your lead leg after every five to eight steps.

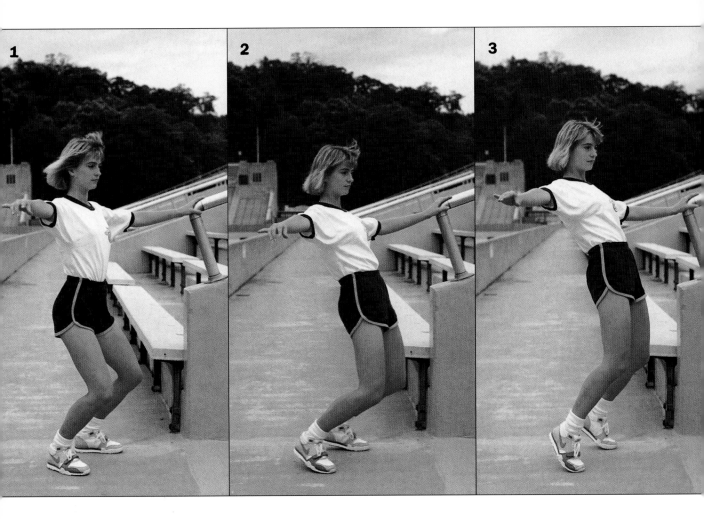

LEG WORKERS *(continued)*

SISSY SQUATS This exercise is quite strenuous despite its name. Stand next to a railing or some other stationary object and extend both arms to your sides, holding the railing with one hand for stability. Bend your knees and drop your pelvis over your heels (1). Straighten your knees and repeat five to eight times. Then bend your knees, drop your pelvis and move it forwards until it is over your toes (2). Keeping your back straight, rock back and forth, shifting the location of your pelvis from over your toes to over your heels five to eight times. Return to a standing position, then bend your knees, move your pelvis until it is over your toes, and straighten your legs while rising on the balls of your feet (3). Continue straightening your legs (4), and return to a standing position (5). Repeat five to eight times.

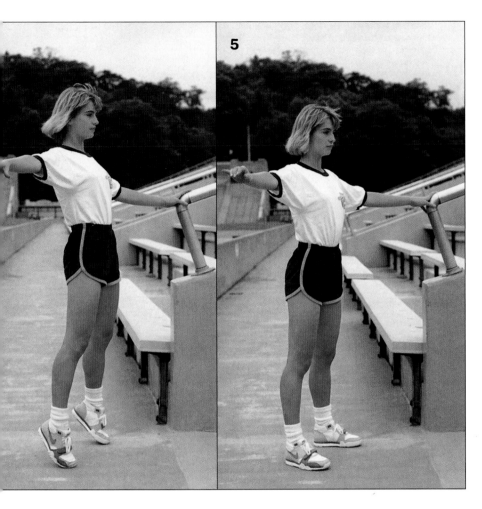

5

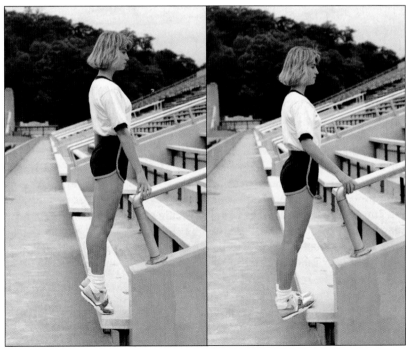

HEEL RAISES Stand on the balls of your feet at the edge of a bench or stadium seat. Hold on to a railing or some other stationary object. Lift your heels *(right)*, and then lower them 20 times. Then drop your heels below the level of the seat *(far right)*, and hold this calf muscle stretch for 30 seconds. Repeat the sequence twice.

RUNG SERIES Warm up with 100 jumping jacks, then jump up to hang from the first rung of a horizontal ladder. Perform two pull-ups *(right)*. Move forwards three rungs *(centre)*, then perform two more pull-ups. Continue in this manner until you reach the end of the ladder. Perform two final pull-ups, and then three to five bent-knee leg lifts *(far right)*.

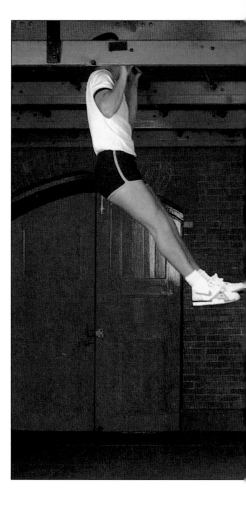

Horizontal Ladder Circuit

In order to perform this series of exercises, you must have access to a playground area or a gym with a horizontal ladder setup. Although children love to use horizontal ladders for play, this equipment can be a powerful conditioner for grip strength and the muscles of your forearms, upper arms, the hip flexor muscles and the latissimus dorsi in your back. In addition, you will be deriving some cardiovascular benefit from the jumping jacks in this mini-circuit. In order to perform this circuit correctly, you must be able to do pull-ups. If you have difficulty, a partner can help lift you.

You can traverse the horizontal ladder in two ways — either by gripping each horizontal rung one after the other in the traditional method or by gripping the side piece and moving hand over hand. The sequence shown on this and the facing page illustrates the horizontal-rung series, while pages 120 and 121 show the sidepiece series.

When you perform this circuit, alternate the rung and sidepiece series twice. Perform eight to 10 pull-ups on one pass across the bars, unless the number of horizontal rungs limits you to six pull-ups on each pass. If this is the case, increase the number of pull-ups you perform at the beginning or the end of each pass.

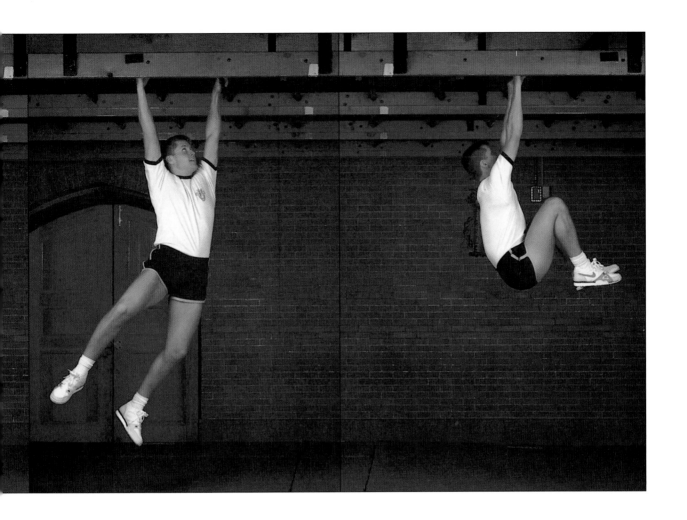

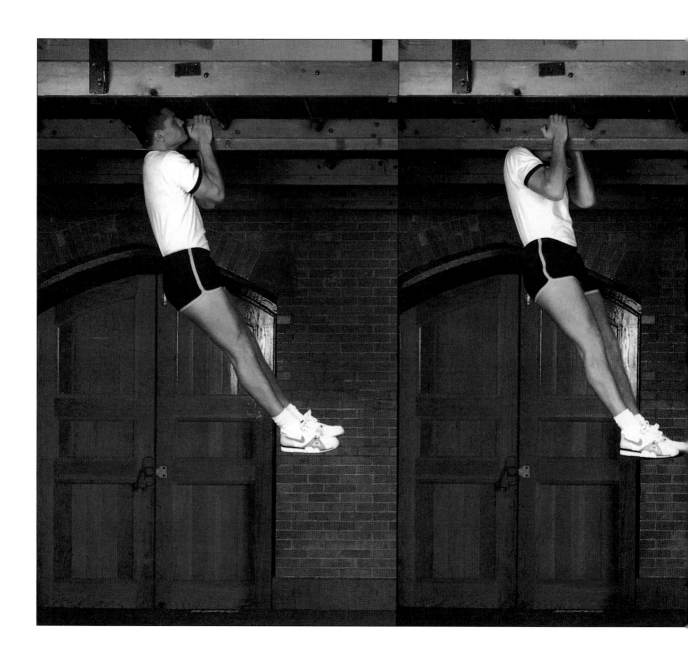

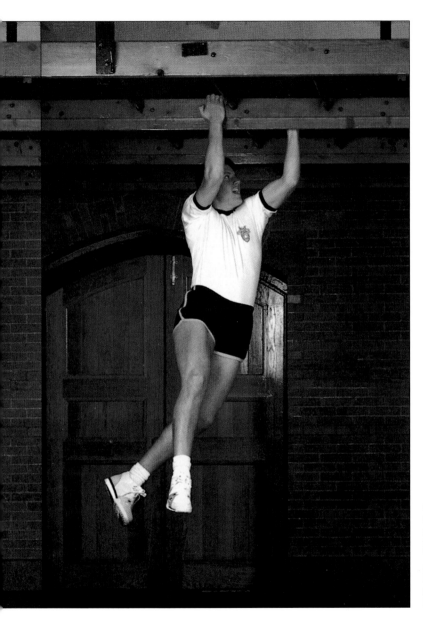

SIDEPIECE SERIES Jump up and hold on to one of the parallel bars with both hands and perform three to five pull-ups, bringing your left ear to the sidepiece *(far left)*. Then do three to five pull-ups to your right ear *(centre)*. Traverse the sidepiece hand over hand *(left)*. At the end of the support, do three to five more left and right-ear pull-ups.

Two-for-One Callisthenics

Most of the exercise sets in this circuit condition two body parts at once, hence the name. The title has a double meaning, since you will also be performing these activities at a certain beat that involves a slow count and half counts. These particular exercises are best done at a tempo of 120 beats per minute; you can listen to music. Count the beats — two per second — to yourself.

Pace yourself as follows. When you do the push-ups, start in the up position and lower yourself, allowing two counts. Then go up for two counts. Now double your time so that you lower yourself on the next count — five — and push up on six. Then come down on seven and push up on eight. On the count of eight, you should have completed three push-ups, one of them slowly and the other two quickly. Perform three more sequences consisting of eight counts each — for nine more push-ups and a total of 32 counts — and then progress to the next activity.

Do all the exercises on these two pages, and then repeat the push-ups to finish the circuit. Four 32-count exercises comprise one set. Perform one or two more sets as you become stronger. As an alternate Two-for-One series, you can perform the movements on pages 124-127. As an advanced Two-for-One, you can combine the exercises on these two pages with those that follow. The alternates are particularly strenuous; do not attempt them unless your abdominals are strong.

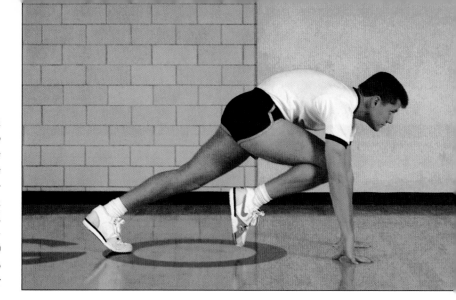

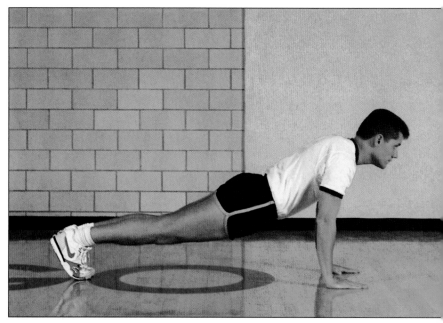

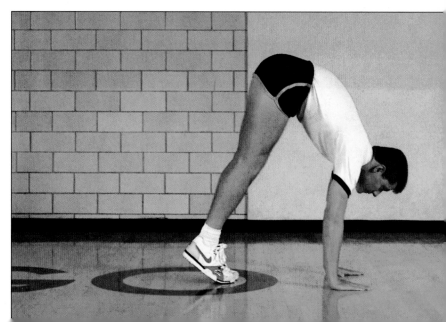

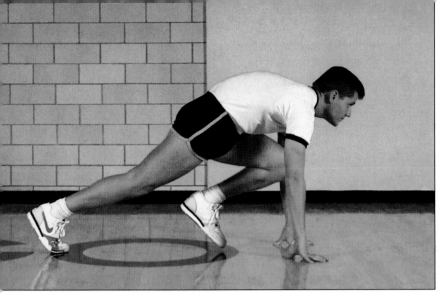

MOUNTAIN CLIMBER Place your hands on the floor shoulder-width apart and extend your legs behind you. Without touching your right foot on the floor, draw your right knee to your chest *(far left)*. Return your right leg to the extended position and then raise your left knee *(left)*.

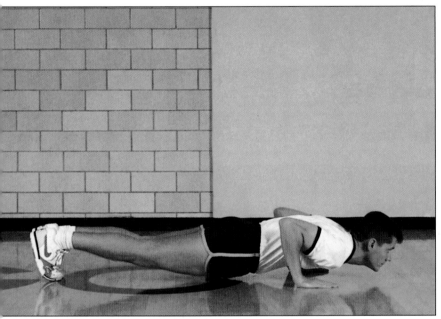

PUSH-UPS From the mountain climber, keep your arms straight and flatten your palms on the floor. Extend both legs and keep your back straight *(far left)*. Bend your elbows and lower your chest to a few centimetres off the floor *(left)*.

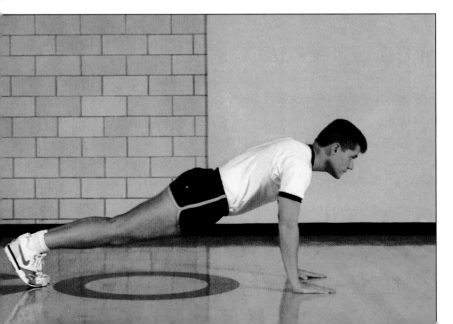

BOTTOMS UP From the extended push-up position, thrust forwards with your toes and lift your buttocks up so that the bottom of your spine points towards the ceiling *(far left)*. Jump back with your toes to the starting position *(left)*. Avoid arching your back. Repeat the push-ups.

123

Two-for-One Alternates

CRAB PUSH-UPS Sit on the floor and raise yourself up on your feet and hands, with fingers pointing to your heels. Lift your chest and pelvis up and keep your elbows extended *(right)*. Drop your body towards the floor by bending your elbows *(far right)*.

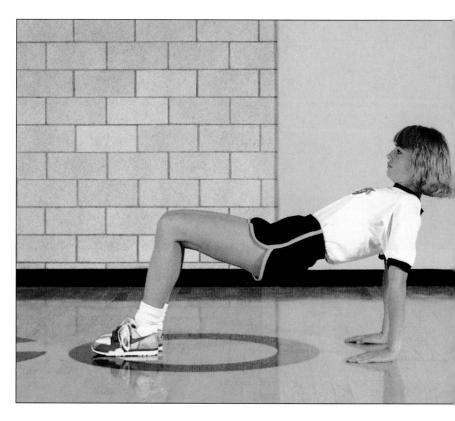

BICYCLE Sit on the floor with your legs extended and your fingers intertwined behind your head. Bring your left knee up and swing your right elbow to meet it *(right)*. Extend your left knee and draw up your right knee, meeting it with your left elbow *(far right)*. Do not arch your back.

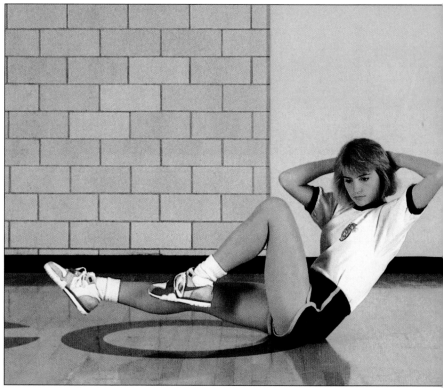

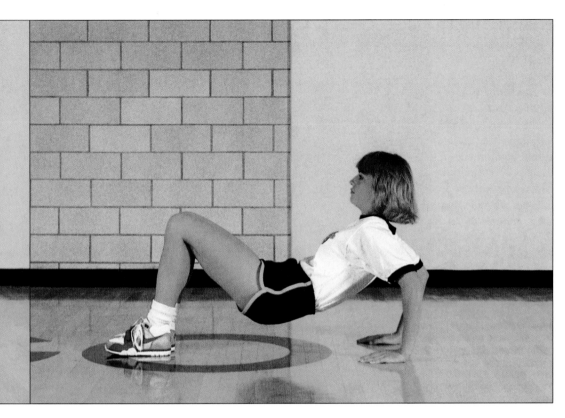

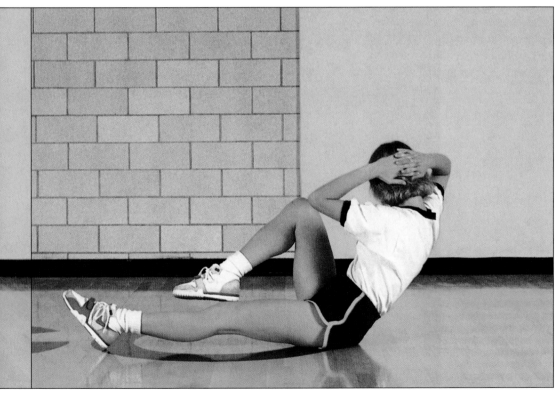

TWO-FOR-ONE ALTERNATES
(continued)

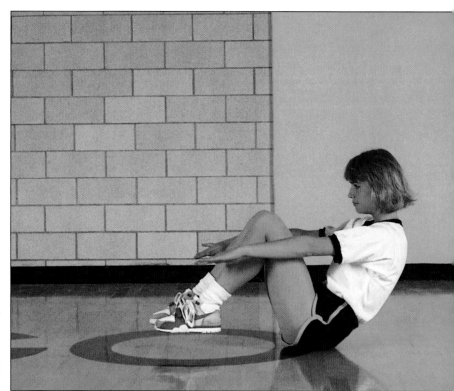

ROW Sit with both knees drawn up, feet off the floor and your arms extended parallel to the floor in front of you *(right)*. Pull your arms back as if you were rowing a boat, and extend your legs *(far right)*. Do not arch your back. Avoid this exercise if you suffer from lower back pain.

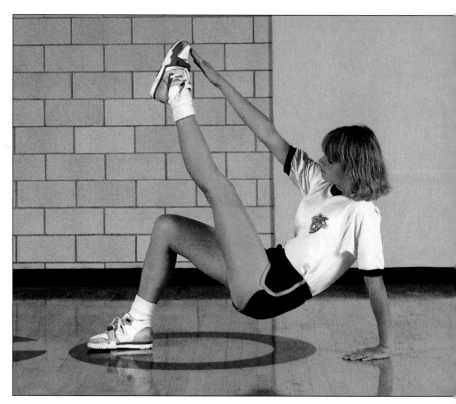

DIAGONAL TOE TOUCH Supported by your hands and feet, lift your pelvis off the floor. Extend your left foot towards the ceiling and touch your toes with your right hand *(right)*. Return your foot and hand to the floor, then extend your right foot towards the ceiling and touch your toes with your left hand *(far right)*.

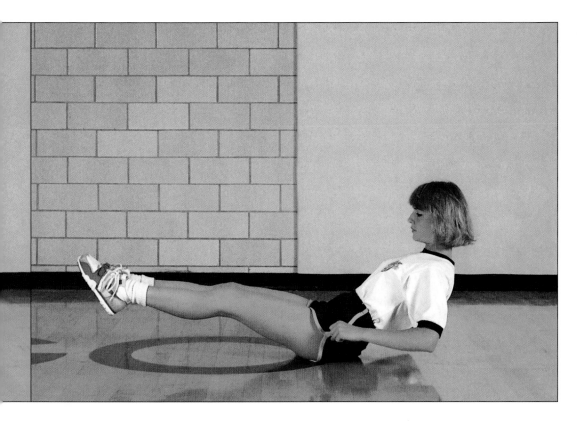

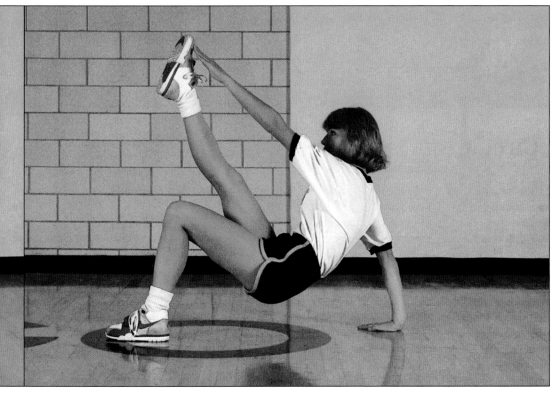

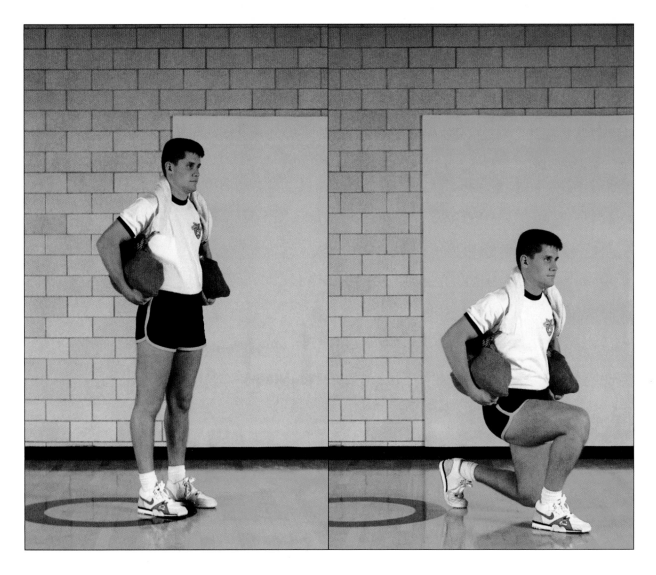

Sandbag Circuit

This circuit contains a number of resistance-training exercises similar to lifting weights. To perform this series, you need some burlap bags filled with sand. Using sandbags is convenient and makes it easy to adjust the weight as you increase your strength. You can fill bags and weigh them on scales. Men may fill two bags each for 12, 14 and 18 or 20 kilograms. Women may fill two bags each for 6, 9 and 12 kilograms. Experiment to find the most appropriate resistance for each exercise.

In addition to the exercises shown here, you can add several more. Perform curls, on pages 106-107, with a sandbag on your chest. You can also do side lateral raises by holding sandbags at your sides and raising them until your arms are parallel to the floor, or biceps curls, which involve bending your elbows.

Perform each exercise continuously for one minute. Then run double time on the spot for one minute before moving on to the next exercise. Finish with a double-time run and start the circuit over again.

LUNGE Attach a rope to two heavy sandbags and wrap a towel around the rope so that you can drape it comfortably over your shoulders. Stand erect and hold the sandbags to keep them steady *(above, left)*. Take one step forwards with your right foot and drop down so that your left knee comes within two centimetres of the floor *(above)*. Return to the starting position by pushing off the right foot. Repeat on your left leg.

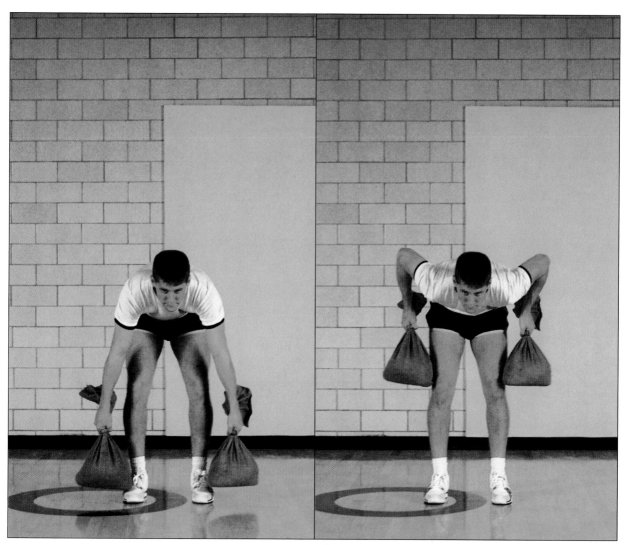

BEND-OVER ROW Hold two moderate to heavy sandbags at your sides, keep your knees bent slightly, and bend over so that the sandbags are several centimetres off the floor *(above, left)*. Lift the sandbags until your hands are at hip level *(above)*. Return to the starting position. Avoid this exercise if you suffer from lower back pain.

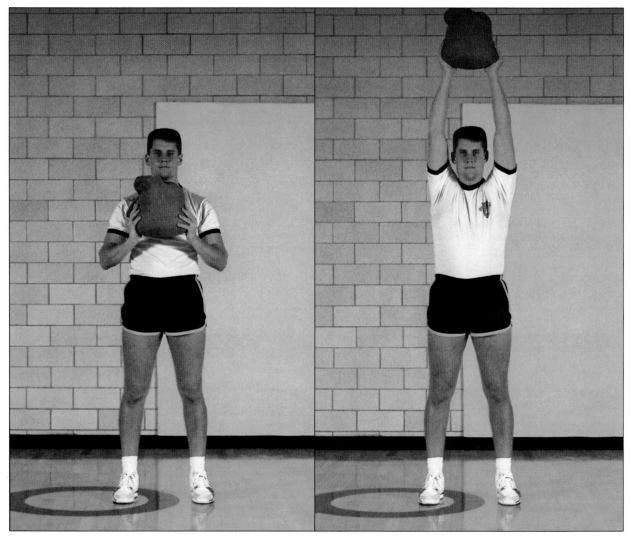

MILITARY PRESS Stand with your feet apart and your knees bent slightly, holding a sandbag in front of you at chest level *(above, left)*. Lift the sandbag directly over your head *(above)*. Avoid arching your back. Return to the starting position.

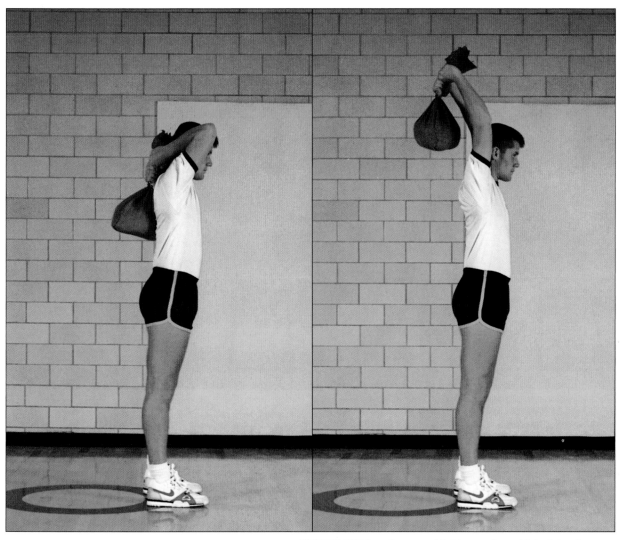

TRICEPS LIFT Stand erect and hold a sandbag with both hands over and behind your head so that the sandbag hangs behind your back *(above, left)*. Extend your arms and lift the sandbag directly up *(above)*. Avoid arching your back. Return to the starting position.

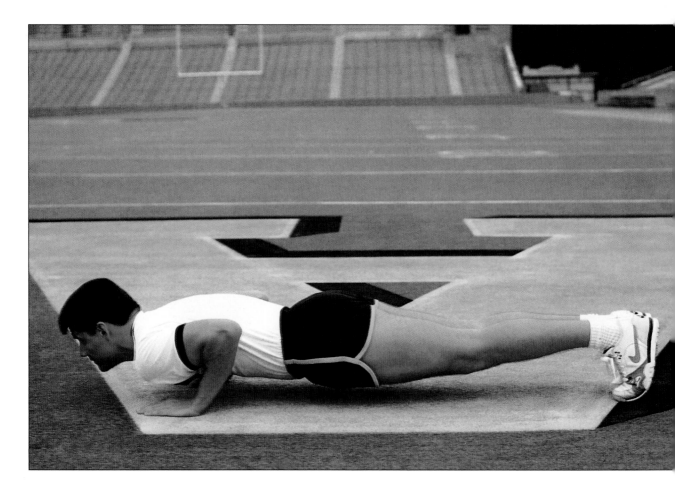

Push-Up Circuit

The push-up is an effective upper body conditioner, particularly for building upper arm, shoulder and chest muscle strength and endurance. Push-ups also help develop strength in your abdominal muscles and lower back, since these areas help to stabilize you while you perform this exercise.

In addition to the classic push-up, for which you place your hands on the ground directly beneath your shoulders, there are a number of variations that help target particular muscles. The push-up on this and the facing page shows proper posture in the up and down positions for the three push-up variations shown on pages 133-135. The push-up circuit continues on pages 136-137, but with different postures — the piked and crab variations.

You can add this upper body mini-circuit to almost any workout. Unless otherwise directed, perform each type of push-up repeatedly for 30 seconds without any rest before progressing to the next push-up.

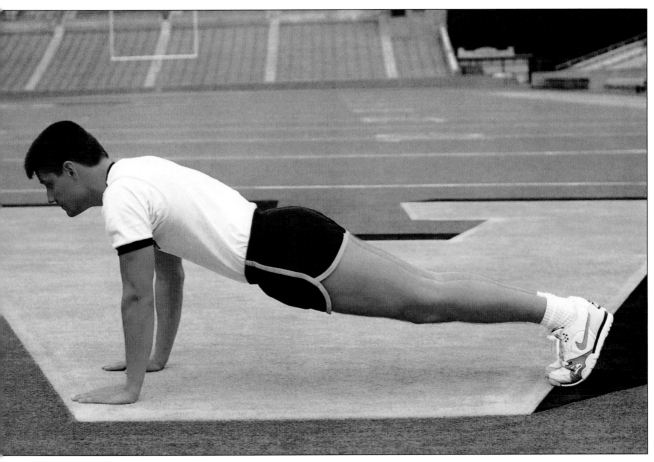

In the down push-up position, keep your hands flat on the ground, your chest a few centimetres above it, and your body and head aligned *(opposite)*. As you push up, extend your arms but do not lock your elbows, keeping your back straight *(above)*.

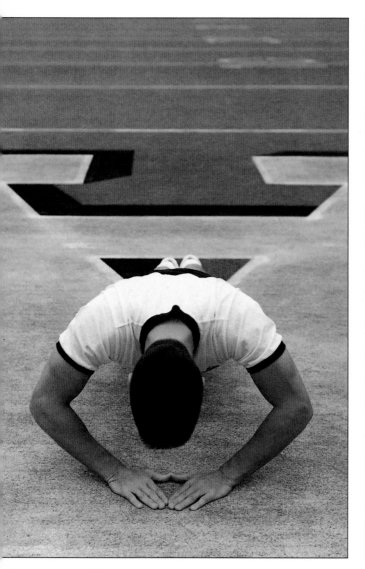

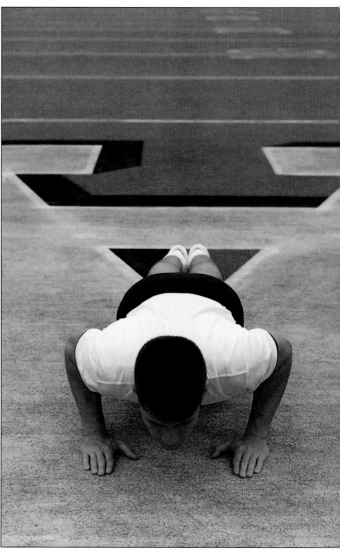

PUSH-UP CIRCUIT (*continued*)

Perform the diamond push-up by placing your hands on the ground so that your thumbs and forefingers form a diamond *(above, left)*. Next do a narrow-grip push-up with your hands placed under your shoulders *(above)*. Then perform a wide-grip push-up with your hands wider than your shoulders *(right)*.

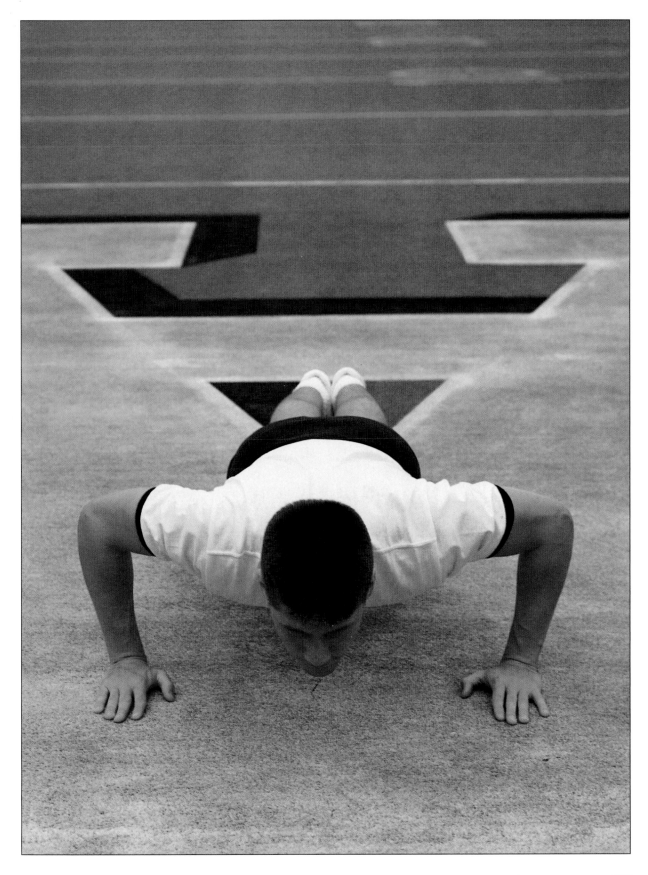

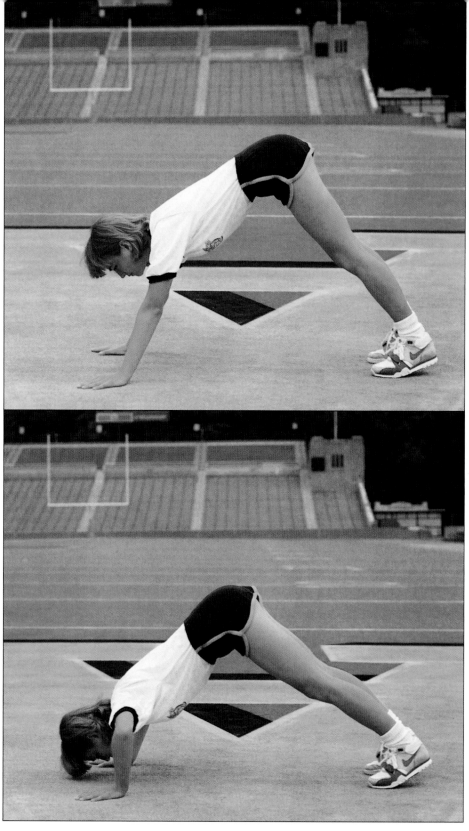

PIKED PUSH-UPS Bend at the hip and make your body into a bridge *(top)*. Making sure you keep your body bent at the same angle, slowly lower yourself until your nose comes within a few centimetres of the ground *(above)*.

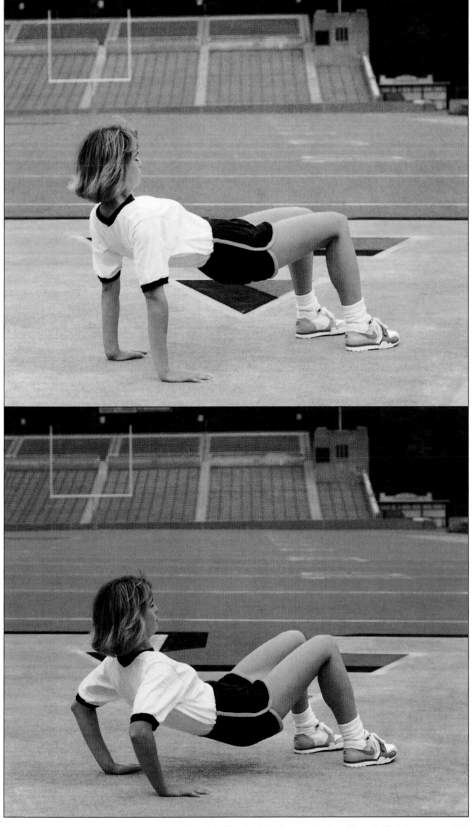

CRAB PUSH-UPS With your feet and hands flat, lift your pelvis up until you are parallel to the ground *(top)*. By bending your arms, lower yourself to within about 10 centimetres of the ground *(above)*. Do as many as you can in 15 seconds.

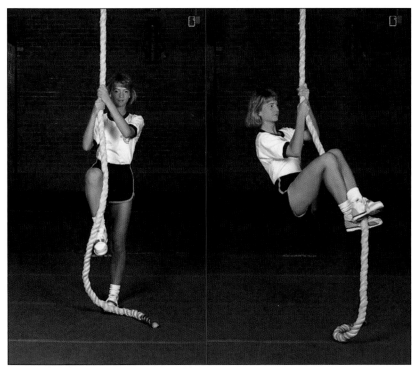

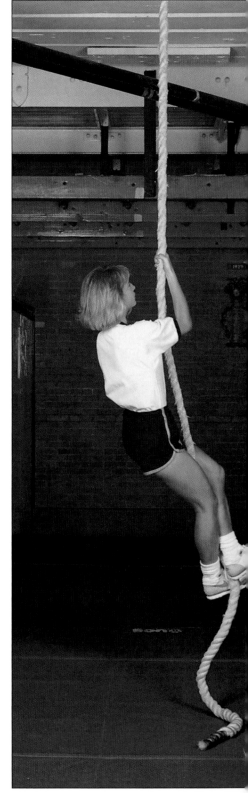

THE CLINCH Grip the rope with both hands at about face level and raise your right foot up so that the rope rests against the inside of your knee and the outside of your foot *(above, left)*. Holding yourself in place with your hands, lift your left leg up and cross your feet to squeeze the rope between your thighs, just above your knees, and the outside edges of your shoes. Hang on the rope in a sitting position *(above, right)*.

Rope Climbing

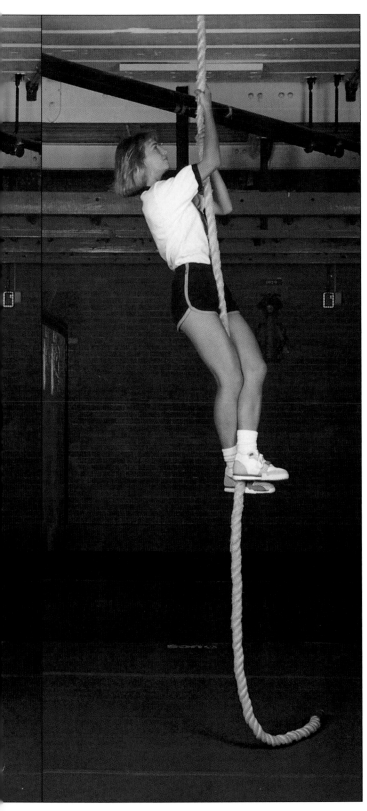

Because it is sometimes essential in combat situations or during troop manoeuvres, rope climbing has long been a staple of military training. Although not often included in non-military fitness programmes, climbing is a superb whole-body muscle strengthener — an effective conditioner for anyone. Not only does it strengthen your upper arms and hand grip, but it conditions your abdominal muscles and thighs as well. Most hemp ropes are too thin and rough for comfortable climbing, but many school and college gyms have rope apparatus made for climbing.

Safety on the ropes is crucial. Always set up mats under the rope. If you are a climbing novice, make sure you have a spotter, and do not climb more than 2 metres off the ground. Begin by climbing slowly until you have mastered the technique, then perform repeat rope climbs until you have climbed a total of 15 to 20 metres.

ASCENDING Keep the rope squeezed between your thighs and shoes. Extend your legs forwards so that you feel as if you are stepping on the rope. Walk your hands up the rope as you extend your legs *(far left)*. To continue, hold the rope tightly with your hands but relax the grip of your thighs and feet. Slide your thighs and feet up until you reach the sitting position again, then clinch. Walk up the rope with your hands and extend your legs until your body is straight *(left)*.

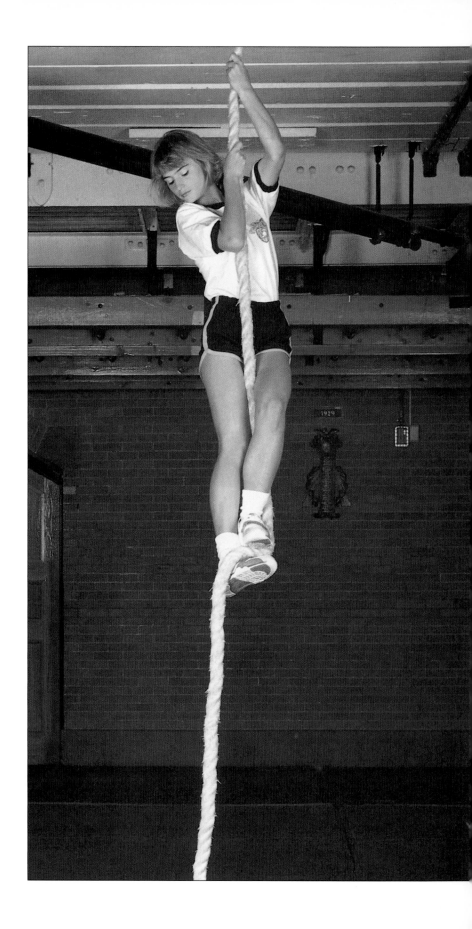

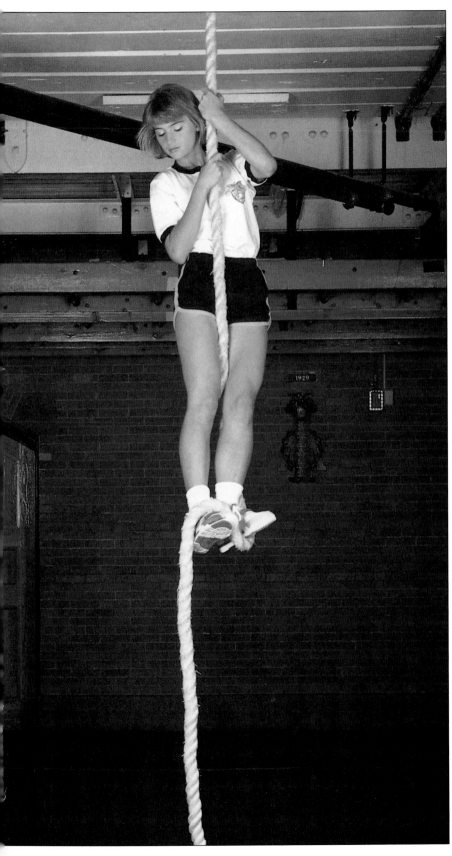

ROPE CLIMBING
(continued)

DESCENDING Once you have reached the top of your climb, lock your feet. From the clinch, drag your left heel across the top of your right foot, with the rope squeezed between them *(far left)*. The rope will loop between your feet so that if you squeeze your feet together, you will be firmly locked in place. Release just enough tension between your feet so that you can slide down the rope under control by walking down hand under hand *(left)*.

ACKNOWLEDGEMENTS

The editors wish to thank Norma MacMillan.

Nutritional analyses provided by Hill Nutrition Associates, New York State.

Index prepared by Ian Tucker.

PHOTOGRAPHY CREDITS

Exercise photography by Andrew Eccles.

ILLUSTRATION CREDITS

Pages 9, 10, 13, illustrations: David Flaherty.

INDEX